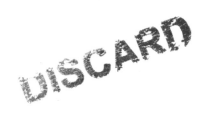

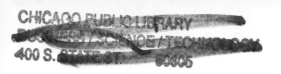

Homelessness, Health, and Human Needs

Committee on Health Care
for
Homeless People

INSTITUTE OF MEDICINE

NATIONAL ACADEMY PRESS
Washington, D.C. 1988

National Academy Press ● **2101 Constitution Avenue, NW** ● **Washington, DC 20418**

NOTICE: The project that is the subject of this report was approved by the Governing Board of the National Research Council, whose members are drawn from the councils of the National Academy of Sciences, the National Academy of Engineering, and the Institute of Medicine. The members of the committee responsible for the report were chosen for their special competences and with regard for appropriate balance.

This report has been reviewed by a group other than the authors according to procedures approved by a Report Review Committee consisting of members of the National Academy of Sciences, the National Academy of Engineering, and the Institute of Medicine.

The Institute of Medicine was chartered in 1970 by the National Academy of Sciences to enlist distinguished members of the appropriate professions in the examination of policy matters pertaining to the health of the public. In this, the Institute acts under both the Academy's 1863 congressional charter responsibility to be an adviser to the federal government and its own initiative in identifying issues of medical care, research, and education.

The work on which this publication is based was performed pursuant to Contract No. 240-86-0073 with the Health Resources and Services Administration of the Department of Health and Human Services. Additional support for this study was contributed by the Veterans Administration and the National Research Council (NRC) Fund. The NRC Fund is a pool of private, discretionary, nonfederal funds that is used to support a program of Academy-initiated studies of national issues in which science and technology figure significantly. The NRC Fund consists of contributions from a consortium of private foundations including the Carnegie Corporation of New York, the Charles E. Culpeper Foundation, the William and Flora Hewlett Foundation, the John D. and Catherine T. MacArthur Foundation, the Andrew W. Mellon Foundation, the Rockefeller Foundation, and the Alfred P. Sloan Foundation; the Academy Industry Program, which seeks annual contributions from companies that are concerned with the health of U.S. science and technology and with public policy issues with technology content; and the National Academy of Sciences and the National Academy of Engineering endowments.

Library of Congress Cataloging-in-Publication Data
Institute of Medicine (U.S.). Committee on Health Care for Homeless
People.
   Homelessness, health, and human needs / Committee on Health Care
for Homeless People, Institute of Medicine.
      p.   cm.
   Includes bibliographies and index.
   ISBN 0-309-03835-9. ISBN 0-309-03832-4 (pbk.)
   1. Homelessness—Health aspects—United States. 2. Poor—Medical
care—United States.   I. Title.
   [DNLM: 1. Delivery of Health Care—United States. 2. Health
Services Accessibility—United States. 3. Homeless persons.   WA
300 I59h]
RA770.I46 1988
362.1'08806942—dc19
DNLM/DLC   8-25466
for Library of Congress   CIP

Cover art by John Jenkins, a free-lance artist working in New York City, whose experience as a homeless man in the shelter system provided the basis for this drawing. Reprinted, with permission, from *Working with Homeless People: A Guide for Staff and Volunteers* (rev. ed.), Amy Haus, editor. New York City: Columbia University Community Services, 1988.

Committee on Health Care for Homeless People

BRUCE C. VLADECK (*Chairman*),* President, United Hospital Fund of New York, New York City

DREW ALTMAN, Commissioner, New Jersey Department of Human Services, Trenton

ELLEN L. BASSUK, Associate Professor of Psychiatry, Harvard Medical School

WILLIAM R. BREAKEY, Associate Professor, Department of Psychiatry and Behavioral Sciences, Johns Hopkins University

A. ALAN FISCHER,* Professor and Chairman, Department of Family Medicine, Indiana University School of Medicine

CHARLES R. HALPERN,* Professor of Law, City University of New York Law School at Queen's College

JUDITH R. LAVE, Professor, Department of Economics, University of Pittsburgh

JACK A. MEYER, President, New Directions for Policy, Washington, D.C.

GLORIA SMITH, Commissioner, Michigan Department of Public Health, Lansing (currently Dean, College of Nursing, Wayne State University)

LOUISA STARK, Adjunct Professor, Department of Anthropology, Arizona State University

NATHAN STARK,* Kominers, Fort, Schlefer and Boyer, Washington, D.C.

MARVIN TURCK, Associate Dean and Professor of Medicine, University of Washington, and Medical Director, Harborview Medical Center, Seattle

PHYLLIS WOLFE, Executive Director, Robert Wood Johnson/Pew Memorial Trust Health Care for the Homeless Project, Washington, D.C.

Study Staff, Division of Mental Health and Behavioral Medicine

ALAN R. SUTHERLAND, Study Director
DEBORAH S. SWANSBURG, Program Officer
JAMES R. BRUNER, Study Secretary/Project Assistant

FREDRIC SOLOMON, Director, Division of Mental Health and Behavioral Medicine
ELIZABETH H. KITSINGER, Division Secretary

---

*Member, Institute of Medicine.

iii

Preface

This study was undertaken at the request of the U.S. Congress as stated in the Health Professionals Training Act of 1985 (P.L. 99-129). The act directed the secretary of the Department of Health and Human Services to arrange with the National Academy of Sciences, through its Institute of Medicine, for a study of the delivery of inpatient and outpatient health care services to homeless people. That provision was one of various legislative initiatives concerning the growing problem of homelessness that the Congress has considered in recent years (see Appendix A). The congressional mandate in P.L. 99-129 was implemented in October 1986, when the Department of Health and Human Services, through its Health Resources and Services Administration, entered into a contract with the Institute of Medicine. Additional funding was provided by the National Research Council and, subsequently, by the U.S. Veterans Administration.

The study was directed at three tasks specified in P.L. 99-129: (1) an evaluation of whether the eligibility requirements in existing health care programs prevent homeless individuals from receiving health care services; (2) an evaluation of the efficiency of the delivery of health care services to homeless individuals; and (3) recommendations for activities by federal, state, local, and private entities that would improve the availability of health care service delivery to homeless individuals.

As in all studies done under the auspices of the National Academy of Sciences, the first step in the process was to select a committee of knowledgeable people to conduct the study. A 13-member panel was drawn from the disciplines of anthropology, economics, epidemiology, family and internal medicine, law, nursing, political science, psychiatry, public administration, and social work. At its initial meeting in December 1986, the Committee on Health Care for Homeless People adopted the following approach for the study.

Recognizing the limitations of the research literature on homeless people, their health problems, and the health services they receive, the committee directed a search of unpublished reports as well as published studies and documents. To supplement the existing literature, the committee commissioned the following 10 papers written by experts on subjects of special concern:

- "Legal Barriers to Access: The Unmet Health Care Needs of Homeless People," Arlene Kanter;
- "A Critique of the Methodologies of Counting the Homeless," Charles Cowan, William Breakey, and Pamela Fischer;
- "Rural Homelessness," Lawrence Patton;
- "The Dynamics of Homelessness," Russell Schutt;
- "Homelessness: A Medical Viewpoint," William Vicic and Patricia Doherty;
- "Shelter and Health Care of Homeless Families, Homeless Children, Homeless Adult Individual Females, and Homeless Battered Women and Their Children," Deborah Reisman Fink;
- "Ancillary Health Care Services for Homeless Persons: Availability and Delivery," Marianne Gleason;
- "Mental Health and the Homeless Population," Andrew Ziegler;
- "Alcohol Problems Among the Contemporary American Homeless Population: An Analytic Review of the Literature," Pamela Fischer; and
- "Illicit Substance Abuse Among the Homeless," Virginia Mulkern.

Significant findings from these papers are incorporated throughout this report; two papers, those on the methodologies of counting the homeless and on the homeless in rural areas, are included as Appendixes B and C, respectively.

The committee regarded both the gaps in data and the desirability of first-hand acquaintance with homelessness as reasons to conduct site visits. Members of the committee, accompanied by Institute of Medicine staff and consultants, visited 11 cities and (with separate funding from the Department of Health and Human Services) rural areas in four states to learn the characteristics of homelessness in those communities and the nature of health services directed to homeless people. These sites were selected not as a representative sample of programs for the homeless but, rather, as potential models of service delivery. At the same time, by interviewing both homeless individuals and people attempting to help the homeless, committee members were able to assess the validity of many findings that appear in the literature.

The committee benefited greatly from the assistance of the national Health Care for the Homeless program of the Robert Wood Johnson Foundation and the Pew Memorial Trust. The directors and staff members of the 19 projects supported by these foundations provided much valuable information for this report. In addition, the Social and Demographic Research Institute of the University of Massachusetts at Amherst, which is under contract with the Robert Wood Johnson and Pew foundations to provide program monitoring and evaluation, generously shared its data and undertook special analyses on the committee's behalf.

This report begins by trying to answer the question, "Who are the homeless?" To dispel myths about homelessness and to provide information about its causes, Chapter 2 discusses the dynamics of homelessness. Chapter 3 describes the health problems of homeless people. Chapter 4 describes the major barriers homeless people encounter in their effort to obtain health care. Chapter 5 examines health care and health-related service programs designed to meet the special needs of homeless people. Chapter 6 summarizes the committee's findings and sets forth its recommendations.

Two aspects of the work of the committee warrant further explanation. First, although the committee's charge was fairly narrow, its examination perforce was fairly broad. Early in the study, the committee determined that the specific aspects of health and health care contained in the congressional charge could not be separated from many aspects of homelessness itself.

The second has to do with the relative amounts of attention, both in the study and in the report, invested in specific health problems and particular subpopulations of the homeless. Reports of studies of some health problems common among homeless people, such as alcoholism or mental illness, are numerous and readily available; these could be summarized rather succinctly. Information on other types of health-related problems, however, often was more anecdotal or based on very recent data, some of which were provided especially for use in this study. Therefore, parts of this report may appear to place greater or lesser emphasis on certain problems than might seem to be warranted by their actual proportion among the hardships of the homeless.

The report, in response to P.L. 99-129, is directed to the United States Congress and to policymakers on the national, state, and local levels, but the committee hopes it will also be of value to those who work directly with the homeless and to the average citizen who has concern for them.

*   *   *   *   *

As chairman of the committee responsible for this report, I want to take this opportunity to thank my colleagues on the committee for their dedication, patience, and extremely hard work on this study. I also wish to acknowledge the many people outside the Institute of Medicine who gave so generously of their time to help enrich our study (see Appendix E). In addition to the authors of commissioned papers listed in the Preface, we take particular note of the contributions of Pamela Fischer of John Hopkins University; Deborah Franklin, a doctoral student in history of science at the University of Pennsylvania; Max Michael of the University of Alabama at Birmingham Medical Center; and James Wright of the University of Massachusetts. I owe a particularly large debt of personal gratitude to Susan Neibacher, director of the New York City Health Care for the Homeless Program at the United Hospital Fund, who generously served, with her customary great patience and tolerance, as my personal guide through the thicket of issues the committee encountered on homelessness.

None of these efforts, of course, would have produced a report without the intensive labors of a dedicated professional staff at the Institute of Medicine, especially the study director, Alan Sutherland, and his deputy, Deborah Swansburg. An especially large thank you is owed to their supervisor, Fredric Solomon, director of the Division of Mental Health and Behavioral Medicine, and to the Institute's Associate Executive Officer for Programs, Marian Osterweis.

BRUCE C. VLADECK, *Chairman*
Committee on Health Care for
Homeless People

Contents

APPENDIXES

Homelessness,
Health,
and Human Needs

1   Who Are the Homeless?

INTRODUCTION

There have always been homeless people in the United States. As economic circumstances and demographic forces have fluctuated, so have the size and composition of the homeless population, although relatively permanent skid rows where homeless people congregate have long been a feature of many large cities.

In the past decade, however, the problem of homelessness has increasingly captured public attention. Not only has the number of homeless people increased dramatically within the last several years but the composition of the homeless population has also changed appreciably during that period: For example, middle-aged men make up a shrinking fraction of all homeless people, and families with young children are the fastest growing component of the homeless population (U.S. Conference of Mayors, 1987). Growing public awareness of homelessness is also connected to changes in the geographic dispersion of homeless people, who are becoming more visible in neighborhoods and communities that would not have imagined their presence in the past.

This chapter briefly describes homelessness in the United States. It begins by defining homelessness, assessing methodologies used to count homeless people, and reviewing recent scholarly literature on the subject. The chapter continues by examining the socio-demographic characteristics of homeless people, with emphasis on adult individuals, families and children, runaway and throwaway youths,* the elderly, and people in

---

* "Throwaway" youths refers to children and adolescents who are evicted from their homes by their parents or another adult in a position of responsibility for them.

1

rural areas. In the course of this discussion the issues relating to the prevalence of health and mental health problems inevitably arise, but these are reviewed in greater detail in Chapter 3, Health Problems of Homeless People.

DEFINITION OF HOMELESS

For the purpose of this report, the definition of homeless or homeless person is the same as that in P.L. 100-77, the Stewart B. McKinney Homeless Assistance Act, enacted in July 1987 (U.S. Congress, House, 1987):

(1) an individual who lacks a fixed, regular, and adequate nighttime residence; [or]

(2) an individual who has a primary nighttime residence that is—

(A) a supervised or publicly operated shelter designed to provide temporary living accommodations (including welfare hotels, congregate shelters, and transitional housing for the mentally ill);

(B) an institution that provides a temporary residence for individuals intended to be institutionalized; or

(C) a public or private place not designed for, or ordinarily used as, a regular sleeping accommodation for human beings.

This definition refers specifically to homeless individuals, but it is equally applicable to homeless families.

COUNTING THE HOMELESS

Even within the framework of a relatively straightforward definition, there is considerable uncertainty about the number of people who are homeless at any given time in the United States. Conventional methods of enumerating populations, such as the census, are based upon counting people where they live. Not only do people move in and out of homelessness but the methodological problems involved in counting people without a fixed residence are formidable. Studies that have attempted to count homeless people have been subject to severe criticism. For example, samples are generally small and may not be generalizable to other locales, data are often collected from single sites, samples often are not systematically drawn, measures and definitions of homelessness are inconsistent, and the rural population is virtually unidentified. For all these reasons, the various studies cannot be easily compared or generalized. (Appendix B of this report contains a detailed analysis of the three most common methods of counting homeless people and the technical strengths and weaknesses of each.)

TABLE 1-1   National Estimates of the Homeless Population[a]

Source	Estimate	Assumptions Used
Hombs and Snyder (1982)	2,200,000	Based on a small number of high local estimates. Apparently uses city populations to estimate a rate of homelessness. Applies constant rate of homelessness to the entire country.
U.S. Department of Housing and Urban Development (1984)		
1.	192,000	Applies a street-to-shelter ratio to estimates of the sheltered population.
2.	254,000	Based on estimates for 60 cities. Uses metropolitan population as the base. Calculates rates separately for large, medium, and small areas.
3.	586,000	Takes highest local estimates. Uses metropolitan population as the base. Assumes a constant rate of homelessness nationwide.
Tucker (1987)	700,000	Based on estimates for 50 cities. Uses city populations as the base. Allows rates to vary for large, medium, and small cities.
Freeman and Hall (1986)	287,000	Applies a street-to-shelter ratio to estimates of the sheltered population.
Alliance Housing Council (1988)	735,000 on a given night; 1.3 million to 2.0 million during 1988	Based on reinterpretation and extrapolation from U.S. Dept. of Housing and Urban Development (1984) studies. Assumes suburban rate of 1/3rd the city rate. Assumes 20% growth in homelessness each year.

[a]Adapted from Alliance Housing Council (1988).

The range of estimates of the number of homeless people is wide (Table 1-1). At the low end is the U.S. Department of Housing and Urban Development (1984) estimate of 200,000 to 300,000. At the high end are advocates' estimates of more than 2 million (Hombs and Snyder, 1982). Whatever the absolute numbers, the number of homeless people has grown appreciably in recent years. Surveys conducted by the U.S. Conference of Mayors in 25 representative cities in each of the past 2 years identified no city in which the numbers were falling; most cities reported annual increases of 15 to 50 percent (U.S. Conference of Mayors, 1987). A substantial majority of the cities reported that families were the fastest growing component of the homeless population.

One recent estimate of the number of homeless people in the United States, published in June 1988 by the National Alliance to End Homelessness, calculates that currently, on any given night, there are 735,000 homeless people in the United States; that during the course of 1988, 1.3 million to 2.0 million people will be homeless for one or more nights; and that these people are among approximately 6 million Americans who, because of their disproportionately high expenditures for housing costs, are at extreme risk of becoming homeless (Alliance Housing Council, 1988).

For the purposes of this study, the question of precisely how many homeless people there are was not of central importance because homelessness is not a static condition; poor people move in and out of a state of homelessness. Therefore, the committee devoted a major part of its effort to analyzing the composition of the homeless subpopulations and the health-related needs of each group.

STUDIES OF HOMELESSNESS

Since the early 1980s, an extensive body of literature about homeless people has emerged. Although some have described homelessness in the United States impressionistically, a number of scholars have conducted substantial surveys and performed extensive data analyses in order to describe the characteristics of homeless people. The earliest publications on the "new" homeless have focused on the demographic and social characteristics of homeless adults living in large cities, such as New York (Hoffman et al., 1982; Crystal and Goldstein, 1984), Phoenix (Brown et al., 1982, 1983), Portland, Oregon (Multnomah County, Oregon, Department of Human Services, 1984, 1985), Los Angeles (Robertson et al., 1985; Farr et al., 1986), Chicago (Stevens et al., 1983; Rossi et al., 1986), St. Louis (Morse et al., 1985), Milwaukee (Rosnow et al., 1985), Boston (Bassuk et al., 1984), Philadelphia (Arce et al., 1983), and Baltimore (Fischer and Breakey, 1986). Wider in geographic scope are the studies of the states of Ohio (Roth et al., 1985) and Vermont (Vermont Department of Human Services, 1985). Although the sites at which data were collected often differed—shelters, streets, single room occupancy hotels—as did the sampling strategy and operational criteria for studying homelessness, the data collected from these different areas showed surprising similarities.

Research has also been conducted on subpopulations of homeless people as well as on specialized topics related to homelessness. A substantial number of reports have focused on the homeless mentally ill and on homeless people who suffer from alcohol abuse. A much smaller body of literature exists on other health-related issues. In fact, it was only 3 years ago that the first book on this issue, *Health Care of Homeless People* (Brickner et al., 1985), was published; the importance of the issue and the growth in our knowledge are reflected by the fact that the authors already have begun work on the second edition. There is also a growing body of scholarly work on subpopulations, especially homeless families (Bassuk et al., 1986).

Studies on the demographic and social characteristics of the homeless in the United States have almost always been based upon research conducted in urban areas. Except for the Ohio and Vermont reports, which included both urban and nonurban areas, very little has been published on the homeless in suburban and rural communities—except in newspapers (Washington Post, September 27, 1987; New York Times, October 16, 1987). There is a similar, though less pronounced, paucity of information about certain subpopulations among the contemporary homeless, such as the elderly, youths, individual adult women, the physically disabled, the mentally retarded, and those addicted to illicit drugs.

CHARACTERISTICS OF HOMELESS PEOPLE

Homeless people are a diverse and varied group in terms of age, ethnicity, family circumstances, and health problems. Moreover, the characteristics of the homeless population differ dramatically from one community to another. Even the recent increase in homeless families is not uniform throughout the country. Although homeless families headed by women are predominant among the homeless throughout the country, there are many more homeless two-parent families in the West and Southwest than in New York and other large eastern cities (U.S. Conference of Mayors, 1987). Every city has homeless adults, but the demographics are not uniform throughout the country. Most cities report that adult homeless men tend to be long-term residents of the city. However, during a site visit to San Diego, committee members were informed by both public officials and advocates for the homeless that San Diego's adult homeless male population was composed largely of young men from the West and Midwest who had come to the Southwest in search of jobs.

To make the needs of homeless people more understandable, we describe several subgroups separately: individual adult men and women, families with children, youths, the elderly, and people in rural areas.

Homeless Individual Adults

Although families may represent the fastest growing subgroup among the homeless, individual adults still make up the single largest group among the homeless population. The documented characteristics of homeless adult men and women contradict some popular conceptions of what such people are like.

The U.S. Conference of Mayors (1987) reported that individual men made up 56 percent of the homeless population and individual women made up 25 percent. (The remainder are adolescents or families with children.) Of the 25 cities in the study, 7 reported recent increases in the numbers of homeless women. In 1963, homeless women represented only 3 percent of the homeless population (Bogue, 1963). Researchers indicate that a high proportion of homeless women suffer from serious problems including chronic mental illness and pregnancy-related problems (Wright, 1987; Wright and Weber, 1987; Wright et al., 1987). In addition, homeless women are frequently victims of physical assault, especially rape (Brickner et al., 1985).

Individual homeless men and women have an average age of between 34 and 37 (Morse, 1986); this is significantly lower than those found in previous decades. Homeless women are from 2 to 6 years younger (both mean and median) than homeless men (Multnomah County, Oregon, Department of Human Services, 1984; Robertson et al., 1985; Rossi et al., 1986). Reports from several cities indicate that the sheltered male population is younger still and that homeless women appear to be either very young or elderly. This is important because, unless they are disabled, the age of homeless adults in many parts of the country helps to determine their eligibility for entitlements, especially general assistance and Medicaid.

Homeless adults are likely never to have been married. Reported levels range from 40 percent in Portland, Oregon (Multnomah County, Oregon, Department of Human Services, 1984) to 64 percent in New York City (Hoffman et al., 1982). Homeless women are more likely than homeless men to have been married: In the Portland study, only 29 percent of homeless women had never married compared with 44 percent of homeless men. Never-married homeless adults are generally not members of households and often lack strong family ties. The absence of family ties removes the possibility of finding shelter with family members.

Minorities are overrepresented among homeless people in the nation's larger cities (Table 1-2). This distribution reflects the overrepresentation of minorities in the poorest strata of American society (Morse, 1986).

The proportion of homeless people with a high school diploma has increased during the past 25 years. For example, in 1963, only 19 percent of homeless people in Chicago had completed high school (Bogue, 1963), compared with 35 percent of the general population of Chicago (U.S. Bureau of the Census, 1963). In 1985, 55 percent of the homeless population in that city were high school graduates (Rossi et al., 1986); the comparable figure for the entire population of Chicago was 56 percent, almost identical to that for the homeless population. While there was a greater divergence between the educational level of homeless and general populations in other cities (Roth et al., 1985; Farr et al., 1986), nationally the proportion of homeless adults with high school diplomas is approximately 45 percent.

Contrary to the fears expressed by public officials that their city may attract increasing numbers of homeless people if they do more to help, several recent studies indicate that the great majority of homeless people have been long-term residents of the city in which they are sheltered (Table 1-3). This was confirmed during the site visits. It was also reported that when a city did attract transients, it was generally not by virtue of its entitlement programs but, rather, because of a favorable economic climate and the possibility of employment. People working directly with the homeless in various cities reported to the committee that transient persons failing to find employment in one city tended not to stay long and soon moved on in search of jobs.

Since the mean age of homeless men is approximately 35, it is not surprising that a large number are Vietnam veterans (Table 1-4). Studies of homeless veterans in Los Angeles (Robertson, 1987) and Boston (Schutt, 1985) indicate that they are older than nonveterans, better educated, and more likely to have been married, factors that normally would indicate greater stability. They also tend to be white, although the percentage of ethnic minorities increases substantially among those who served in Vietnam.

As discussed in detail in Chapter 3, psychiatric problems and alcohol and drug abuse are common among homeless veterans. The Los Angeles and Boston studies both reported higher rates of psychiatric hospitalization than among nonveteran homeless people. The Boston study, as well as a study of homeless veterans in San Francisco (Swords to Plowshares, 1986), reported that veterans were more likely to identify substance abuse as a reason for homelessness. The San Francisco study reported that 45 percent suffered from alcohol abuse (19 percent reporting severe alcohol problems) and 23 percent from drug abuse.

The most recent statistics on homeless veterans come from the Homeless Chronically Mentally Ill outreach program conducted by the Veterans Administration as mandated by P.L. 100-6 (Rosenheck et al., 1987). The program is targeted specifically to mentally ill homeless veterans (and therefore does not present a valid sample of all homeless

TABLE 1-2 Ethnic Background of Homeless Adult Individuals (in percent) Compared with That of the General Population

City (Source)	White	Black	Hispanic	Native American	Other	Blacks as Percentage of General Population[a]	Native Americans as Percentage of General Population[a]
New York (Crystal et al., 1982)[b]	11.0	72.7	15.7		0.6	25.2	0.2
New York (Hoffman et al., 1982)[b]	15.0	64.0	21.0		1.0	25.2	0.2
Detroit (Mowbray et al., 1985)	25.7	73.0			1.4	63.0	0.3
Chicago (Rossi et al., 1986)	28.9	55.6	4.0	7.1	4.3	39.8	0.2
Baltimore (Clark, 1985)[c]	35.0	62.0			3.0	54.7	0.3
St. Louis (Morse et al., 1985)	35.1	64.9				45.5	0.1
Chicago (Stevens et al., 1983)	41.0	56.0	1.0	2.0		39.8	0.2

Los Angeles (Robertson et al., 1985)	51.0	30.0	11.0	6.0	3.0	17.0	0.5
Milwaukee (Rosnow et al., 1985)	60.0	32.0	4.0	4.0		23.0	0.7
Phoenix (Brown et al., 1983)	61.0	9.0	17.0	12.0	2.0	4.8	1.4
Ohio (Roth et al., 1985)	65.3	29.8	3.4		0.6	9.9	0.1
Portland (Multnomah County, Oregon, 1985)[c]	73.0	11.0		10.0		7.5	0.9
Portland (Multnomah County, Oregon, 1984)	77.0	6.0	4.0	10.0	1.0	7.5	0.9

NOTE: Hispanic populations could not be compared because of the inconsistency of definitions.

[a]Source of general population data: U.S. Bureau of the Census (1980).
[b]Men only.
[c]Women only.

veterans), but it is both the most recent research on homeless veterans and the most geographically comprehensive. The outreach effort was conducted in 26 states and included Veterans Administration medical centers serving rural, suburban, and urban areas. In its first 4 months of operation (May–September 1987) the program made contact with 6,342 homeless veterans.

Of the veterans contacted, 98.6 percent were men; 1.4 percent were women. The average age was 43; 75 percent were either divorced or had never married. Sixty percent were white, 30 percent were black, and 9 percent were Hispanic. In regard to education, 82 percent were high school graduates. Thirty percent had served in combat, and 1.7 percent had been prisoners of war; 9 percent were diagnosed as having combat-related posttraumatic stress disorder. With regard to the time of their military duty, 38 percent were veterans of the Vietnam era, 21 percent served in the post-Vietnam period, and 18 percent served in the period between the Korean and Vietnam conflicts. Only 9 percent served in World War II and 10 percent in Korea.

Several authors have reported that between 5 and 10 percent of the homeless are employed full-time and between 10 and 20 percent are employed part-time or episodically (Brown et al., 1982, 1983; Multnomah County, Oregon, Department of Human Services, 1984, 1985; Rossi et al., 1986). These people frequently perform unskilled labor; are on the bottom rung of the economic ladder; and often lack job security, health insurance, and the skills necessary to succeed in a high-tech economy.

TABLE 1-3   Length of Residency of Homeless Adult Individuals

City or State	Percent	No. of Years	Source
New York City[a]	82	≥5	Crystal et al. (1982)
Los Angeles[b]	74	≥2	Robertson et al. (1985)
New York City[a]	75	≥5	Hoffman et al. (1982)
Chicago	72.3	≥10	Rossi et al. (1986)
Milwaukee	71	≥1	Rosnow et al. (1985)
Los Angeles[a]	64.5	≥1	Farr et al. (1986)
Ohio	63.5	≥1	Roth et al. (1985)
Baltimore	60	≥10	Fischer et al. (1986)
Portland	59	≥2	Multnomah County, Oregon (1984)

[a]Men only.

[b]The 10.5 percent differential between the studies by Robertson et al. (1985) and Farr et al. (1986) in Los Angeles can be accounted for based on the populations sampled. Robertson and colleagues sampled the downtown skid row *and* the Venice Beach/Santa Monica areas; Farr and colleagues sampled only the downtown skid row area.

TABLE 1-4   Homeless Veterans

City (Source)	Percentage of Homeless Men Sampled Who Are Veterans	Vietnam-Era Veterans as Percentage of Homeless Veterans
Baltimore (Fischer et al., 1986)	51	35
Boston (Schutt, 1985)	37	
Los Angeles (Robertson et al., 1985)	47	33
Los Angeles (Farr et al., 1986)	33	43
Net York City (Crystal et al., 1982)	32	
Detroit (Solarz and Mowbray, 1985)	36	16

Many are homeless because their incomes have not kept pace with the dramatic increase in housing costs. The loss of a day or two of pay may make the difference between paying rent and being evicted.

Homeless Families

As mentioned previously, the fastest growing subgroup among the homeless population consists of families with children. In late 1986, the U.S. Conference of Mayors estimated that such families made up 28 percent of all homeless people in the 25 cities participating in the conference's annual survey of hunger, homelessness, and poverty in America. Most homeless families are headed by women with two or three children (Bassuk et al., 1986). Most of the children are under the age of 5 and are spending their critical developmental years without the stability and security of a permanent home (Towber, 1986a,b; Bassuk and Rubin, 1987; Wright and Weber, 1987).

The literature on the characteristics and needs of homeless families is largely anecdotal, although there are a few systematic studies describing the status and unmet needs of homeless families and the health status (Wright and Weber, 1987), emotional problems (Bassuk et al., 1986; Bassuk and Rubin, 1987; Bassuk and Gallagher, in press; Boxill and Beatty, in press), nutritional status (Acker et al., 1987), and problems in education and learning (Bassuk et al., 1986; Bassuk and Rubin, 1987) of homeless children. To date, the findings are generally descriptive, and there are large regional differences; only a few attempts have been made to generate and test hypotheses about the antecedents, course, and consequences of family homelessness by studying appropriate comparison groups. Despite limitations of the data base, reports of shelter providers, clinicians, agencies, advocates, and policymakers (Simpson et al., 1984; Gallagher, 1986), as well as the committee's site visits to sheltering facilities, tend to support the findings of existing studies. The combined information allows for some generalizations about the characteristics and needs of homeless families.

The vast majority of homeless families are headed by women, but the percentages vary by region. In western regions there are more intact homeless families than in eastern regions (Bassuk et al., 1986; Towber, 1986a,b; McChesney, 1986; Dumpson, 1987). Homeless families that include both parents appear to be more common in rural areas than in urban areas (see Appendix C). Because there is a lack of systematic information about the characteristics of intact homeless families, particularly the fathers, the following discussion concentrates primarily on mothers and children.

Homeless mothers tend to be in their late 20s (Bassuk et al., 1986; McChesney, 1986; Towber, 1986a,b; Dumpson, 1987), are either single or divorced, and have completed at least several years of high school (Bassuk et al., 1986; Towber, 1986a,b; Dumpson, 1987). Their ethnic status tends to mirror the ethnic composition of the area where they are living, with minorities overrepresented in the cities and whites predominating in suburban and rural areas (Bassuk et al., 1986). The vast majority of homeless families are recipients of Aid to Families with Dependent Children (AFDC). A Massachusetts study indicated that long-term AFDC users (those receiving benefits for longer than 2 years) are overrepresented among homeless families (Bassuk et al., 1986).

Researchers have reported that homeless mothers typically are quite isolated and have few, if any, supportive relationships. McChesney (1986) studied the support networks of homeless mothers with at least one child who were living in five Los Angeles County family shelters. She described their slide into homelessness as including ". . . many varied and creative means to shelter themselves and their children" in an effort to stave off homelessness. Most striking was the fact that many families could not call on their own parents, brothers, or sisters as resources. There were three major reasons: "either their parents were dead, their parents and siblings didn't live in the Los Angeles area, or their parents and siblings were estranged" (McChesney, 1986). Bassuk and colleagues (1986), in their study of 80 homeless families living in family shelters in Massachusetts, also described fragmented support networks. When asked to name three persons on whom the mothers could depend during times of stress, 43 percent were unable to name anyone or could name only one person, and almost a quarter named their minor child as their principal source of emotional support (Bassuk et al., 1986). In addition to economic and support system factors, serious health problems may also increase a family's risk of becoming homeless.

Many homeless mothers are victims of family violence, which suggests considerable overlap between families residing in family shelters and those residing in battered women's shelters (Ryback and Bassuk, 1986). Generally, a woman fleeing directly from an abusive mate turns to a battered women's shelter rather than to a family shelter. According to Bassuk et al. (1986), 45 percent of the women they interviewed in Massachusetts family shelters had a history of an abusive relationship with a spouse or mate, but this was generally not the immediate cause of their homelessness. In the only study reporting data about probable child abuse, Bassuk and coworkers found that 22 percent of homeless mothers were currently involved in an investigation or follow-up of child neglect or abuse (Bassuk et al., 1986; Bassuk and Rubin, 1987).

Many families had histories of residential instability and moved several times prior to their current shelter stay; most moved within the community where they were sheltered. A majority of families had been doubled up in overcrowded apartments with friends or relatives, while some had previously resided in other shelters or welfare hotels (Bassuk et al., 1986; Towber, 1986a,b).

A substantial proportion of homeless families using the sheltering system can be characterized as multiproblem families (Bassuk et al., 1986). These families have chronic economic, educational, vocational, and social problems; have fragmented support networks; and have difficulty accessing the traditional service delivery system; ". . . these families use a disproportionally large amount of social services and . . . traditional techniques of treating them fail or, at best, are only marginally successful . . . " (Kronenfeld et al., 1980). The multiproblem family typically seeks assistance when a crisis occurs, but ceases contact with the agency when the crisis abates (Gallagher, 1986).

Studies specifically describing the characteristics and needs of homeless children are quite sparse; studies seeking to provide an estimate of the number of homeless children nationwide are nonexistent. However, the magnitude of the problem can be seen in even the most conservative estimates: If there are approximately 735,000 people homeless on any given night (ICF Inc., 1987), and 25 percent of these people are members of intact families (U.S. Conference of Mayors, 1986), of whom 55 percent are children (Barbanel, 1985), then a minimum of 100,000 children are homeless on any given night of the year. This figure includes only children of intact families; it does not include runaway, throwaway, or abandoned children on the streets or in institutions.

Not surprisingly, researchers have reported erratic school attendance among homeless children. Shelters are frequently located far away from a school, and transportation may be lacking. Preliminary data reported by the Traveler's Aid Program and Child Welfare League (1987) indicate that of 163 families with 331 children in eight cities, only 57 percent of the homeless children attended school regularly. A study of 52 families residing in five New York City welfare hotels reported that, according to parents, 60 percent of their children missed less than 3 days of school per month, 30 percent missed between 4 and 10 days of school per month, and 10 percent missed more than 10 days a month, which is over half of the school days (Columbia University Masters of Public Administration Program, 1985).

Homeless Runaway and Throwaway Youths

The amount of systematic data describing the characteristics of homeless adolescents is even scantier than those for other homeless subpopulations. In addition to its site visits, the committee reviewed three recent studies of runaway and throwaway youths:

- the 1985 Greater Boston Adolescent Emergency Network (GBAEN) study (1985) of 84 adolescents using 11 shelters throughout Massachussetts;
- the 1983 study of 118 adolescents in 7 shelters in New York City completed by David Shaffer and Carol L. M. Caton (1984); and
- the 1984 study of 149 adolescents in a crisis center in Toronto, conducted by Mark-David Janus and colleagues (1987) and funded by the U.S. Department of Justice.

Each study identified running away not so much as an event but as a process; adolescents leave home several times (each successive incident being of longer duration than the previous ones) before actually living on the streets. As Shaffer and Caton (1984) reported, "most adolescents start running away some years before they start to use shelters." With regard to throwaway youths, the Boston study found that 17 percent of subjects who had left home for the first time had been "evicted by their parents" (for the entire population in the Boston study, the proportion evicted, including those with multiple running away incidents, was 12 percent). The fundamental issue in trying to determine the extent of the throwaway youth population is to determine the line between a parent forcing a teenager out of the home and a parent creating a situation so intolerable that the youngster has no option but to leave. To quote

Reverend Leonard A. Schneider, executive director of The Emergency Shelter in New York City:

> It is just possible that running away may be an indication of a very healthy mind, and depression may be a very natural response to an intolerable situation. (Community Council of Greater New York, 1984)

Additional issues regarding the throwaway youth population are discussed in successive chapters: the dynamics of the running away process as it relates to homelessness (Chapter 2); the health problems of runaway youths (Chapter 3); and the current state of services for this population (Chapter 5).

Homeless Elderly People

The percentage of elderly people among the homeless population is less than that among the general population. In all but one recently published study, the elderly made up less than 10 percent of the homeless population (Table 1-5). The figure of 19.4 percent reported by Rossi et al. (1986) for the homeless in Chicago is the highest, but it is still low compared with the 29.6 percent elderly for that city's domiciled population. The contrast is even greater in Ohio, where 6.4 percent of the homeless were over age 60, in contrast to 21.7 percent of the population of the state as a whole (Roth et al., 1985). In the skid row area of Los Angeles, 5 percent of the homeless population is over age 61, in comparison with 17 percent domiciled elderly for the entire county (Farr et al., 1986). Nationwide, only 3 percent of the homeless people who presented themselves for care at the Johnson-Pew Health Care for the Homeless projects were over 65, even though 12 percent of the population of the United States is elderly (Wright and Weber, 1987).

Three hypotheses have been proposed to explain the small percentages of elderly homeless. The first suggests that on turning 65, many homeless people become eligible for various entitlements (Social Security, Medicare, senior citizen housing, etc.). It is possible that such programs generate enough income in benefits, lower housing costs, or both that people are able to leave the streets or at least are prevented from becoming homeless to begin with (Wright and Weber, 1987). The second possibility is that homeless people do not survive to old age, because the realities of a homeless existence are so severely debilitating (Wright and Weber, 1987). A 1956 study of men living on Chicago's skid row revealed an annual death rate of 70 per 1,000, in contrast to the national death rate for white men of 11 per 1,000 (Bogue, 1963). However, a third explanation for the small percentage of homeless elderly may be related to sampling. The subjects of most studies are self-selected and include residents of

TABLE 1-5 Elderly Homeless People

| Location (Source) | Age (yr) | Percentage of: | | |
		Men	Women	Both
St. Louis (Morse, 1986)	60+			2.5
Portland (Multnomah County, Oregon, 1985)	55+		4.0	
Los Angeles (Farr et al., 1986)	61+			4.8
Los Angeles (Robertson et al., 1985)	60+			6.0
Milwaukee (Rosnow et al., 1985)	61+			6.0
New York City (Crystal et al., 1982)[a]	60+	6.0		
Ohio (Roth et al., 1985)	60+			6.4
Portland (Multnomah County, Oregon, 1984)	60+			7.0
New York City (Hoffman et al., 1982)[a]	60+	7.0		
Chicago (Stevens et al., 1983)	56+			8.0
Phoenix (Brown et al., 1983)				9.0
Chicago (Rossi et al., 1986)	55+			19.4
United States (Wright, 1987)	65+			3.0

[a]Men only.

shelters, those who appear for medical treatment, people on the streets willing to be interviewed, and the like. The homeless elderly are particularly reluctant to use certain sheltering facilities that they view as dangerous (Coalition for the Homeless/Gray Panthers of New York City, 1984). To quote Joseph Doolin, the director of the Kit Clarke Senior House, which operates the Cardinal Medeiros Day Center for the homeless elderly of Boston, "younger homeless people tend to 'squeeze out' older street people [from the shelters]" (Doolin, 1986). To the extent that the homeless elderly do not participate in various programs for the homeless, they will be underrepresented in most studies.

The Rural Homeless

Since its first meeting, the committee has been concerned with the fact that almost all the scholarly literature describes the urban homeless. Only two studies, the statewide study of Ohio, *Homelessness in Ohio: A Study of People in Need* (Roth et al., 1985), and the statewide study of Vermont, *Homelessness in Vermont* (Vermont Department of Human Services, 1985), begin to address the physical and mental health problems of homeless people living in rural areas. As a result, the committee commissioned a special study of this population. Subsequently, the Health Resources and Services Administration of the U.S. Department of Health and Human Services, in cooperation with the committee, funded a more detailed analysis of this issue. This included site visits to rural areas in Alabama, Mississippi, Minnesota, and South Dakota. The results of this joint effort of the Institute of Medicine and the Department of Health and Human Services are included in Appendix C of this report.

Briefly, the problems of the rural homeless differ from those of their urban counterparts in several important ways. The rural homeless are far less visible than those in the cities; many live with relatives or others who are part of an extended family network. Some are officially domiciled because they pay a nominal token rent for the use of a shack or other substandard form of housing. However, they are even less likely than their urban counterparts to obtain assistance during times of economic or personal crisis. Rural areas do not have the range of social and financial supports available in most urban areas. Often, homeless people migrate to the cities in search of work; when they fail in that effort, they become a part of the growing numbers of homeless people in the cities. Those who stay in rural areas remain hidden until some event causes them to lose their housing, at which point they can be found living in, for example, cars, abandoned buildings, and woods. Even those communities with previously adequate social service systems are finding it increasingly difficult to serve the growing numbers of homeless people, especially in areas where the decline of agriculture, forestry, and mining is severe.

SUMMARY

The homeless population is heterogeneous. While there is considerable controversy about the number of homeless people, there is general agreement that the number is becoming greater as each year passes. As the number increases, so do the complexities of the homelessness problem:

Why do people become homeless? Which interventions can be used to prevent or resolve the state of homelessness? What strategies must be developed to address the long-term issues involved with this problem?

As has been seen in this chapter, there are several subgroups among the general population of homeless people: individual adults, families with children, adolescents and young adults, the elderly, and people in rural areas. While together they all share one common problem—the lack of a stable residence—they each have specific needs.

As will be seen in the next chapter, the long-established system that has traditionally addressed homelessness now finds itself confronted with a seemingly overwhelming set of problems.

REFERENCES

Acker, P. J., A. H. Fierman, and B. P. Dreyer. 1987. An assessment of parameters of health care and nutrition in homeless children. American Journal of Diseases of Children 141(4):388.

Alliance Housing Council. 1988. Housing and Homelessness. Washington, D.C.: National Alliance to End Homelessness.

Arce, A. A., M. Tadlock, and M. J. Vergare. 1983. A psychiatric profile of street people admitted to an emergency shelter. Hospital and Community Psychiatry 34(9):812–817.

Barbanel, J. 1985. Judge bars city from using offices to shelter homeless. New York Times, August 28: A-1.

Bassuk, E. L., and E. Gallagher. In press. The impact of homelessness on families. Journal of Child and Youth Services.

Bassuk, E. L., and L. Rubin. 1987. Homeless children: A neglected population. American Journal of Orthopsychiatry 5(2):1–9.

Bassuk, E. L., L. Rubin, and A. S. Lauriat. 1984. Characteristics of sheltered homeless families. American Journal of Public Health 75(9):1097–1101.

Bassuk, E. L., L. Rubin, and A. Lauriat. 1986. Characteristics of sheltered homeless families. American Journal of Public Health 76(September):1097–1101.

Bogue, D. 1963. Skid Row. Chicago: University of Chicago Press.

Boxill, N., and A. Beatty. In press. An exploration of mother–child interaction among homeless women and their children using a public night shelter in Atlanta, Georgia. Journal of Child and Youth Services.

Brickner, P. W., L. K. Scharer, B. Conanan, A. Elvy, and M. Savarese, eds. 1985. Health Care of Homeless People. New York: Springer-Verlag.

Brown, C. E., R. Paredes, and L. Stark. 1982. The Homeless of Phoenix: A Profile. Phoenix, Ariz.: Phoenix South Community Mental Health Center.

Brown, C. E., S. MacFarlane, R. Paredes, and L. Stark. 1983. The Homeless of Phoenix: Who Are They and What Should Be Done? Phoenix, Ariz.: Phoenix South Community Mental Health Center.

Clark, A. L. 1985. Health care needs of homeless women in Baltimore. Seminar paper submitted to the faculty of the graduate school of the University of Maryland, College Park, in partial fulfillment of the requirements for the master of science degree.

Coalition for the Homeless/Gray Panthers of New York City. 1984. Crowded Out: Homelessness and the Elderly Poor in New York City. New York: Coalition for the Homeless.

Columbia University Masters of Public Administration Program. 1985. Homeless families living in hotels: The provision of publicly supported emergency temporary housing services. Paper prepared for the Human Resources Administration of New York City. New York: Columbia University.

Community Council of Greater New York. 1984. Runaway and Homeless Youth in New York City: Findings from Recent Research, R. L. Leavitt, ed. New York: Community Council of Greater New York.

Crystal, S. M., and M. Goldstein. 1984. The Homeless in New York City Shelters. New York: Human Resources Administration of the City of New York.

Crystal, S. M., M. Goldstein, and R. Levitt. 1982. Chronic and Situational Dependency: Long-Term Residents in a Shelter for Men. New York: Human Resources Administration of the City of New York.

Doolin, J. 1986. Planning for the special needs of the elderly homeless. The Gerontologist 26(3):229–231.

Dumpson, J. R. 1987. A Shelter Is Not a Home. Report of the Manhattan Borough President's Task Force on Housing for Homeless Families. New York: Manhattan Borough President's Task Force on Housing for Homeless Families.

Farr, R. K., P. Koegel, and A. Burnam. 1986. A Study of Homelessness and Mental Illness in the Skid Row Area of Los Angeles. Los Angeles: Los Angeles County Department of Mental Health.

Fischer, P. J., and W. R. Breakey. 1986. Characteristics of the Homeless with Alcohol Problems in Baltimore: Some Preliminary Results. Baltimore: Department of Health Policy and Management, School of Hygiene and Public Health, and Department of Psychiatry and Behavioral Sciences, School of Medicine, The Johns Hopkins University.

Fischer, P. J., W. R. Breakey, S. Shapiro, J. C. Anthony, and M. Kramer. 1986. Mental health and social characteristics of the homeless: A survey of mission users. American Journal of Public Health 76(5):519–524.

Freeman, R. B., and B. Hall. 1986. Permanent Homelessness in America? Working paper no. 2013. Cambridge, Mass.: National Bureau of Economic Research.

Gallagher, E. 1986. No Place Like Home: A Report on the Tragedy of Homeless Children and Their Families in Massachusetts. Boston: Massachusetts Committee for Children and Youth, Inc.

Greater Boston Adolescent Emergency Network. 1985. Ride a Painted Pony on a Spinning Wheel Ride. Boston: Massachusetts Committee for Children and Youth, Inc.

Hoffman, S. F., D. Wenger, J. Nigro, and R. Rosenfeld. 1982. Who Are the Homeless? A Study of Randomly Selected Men Who Use the New York City Shelters. Albany: New York State Office of Mental Health.

Hombs, M. E., and M. Snyder. 1982. Homelessness in America: Forced March to Nowhere. Washington, D.C.: Community for Creative Non-Violence.

Janus, M.-D., A. McCormack, A. W. Burgess, and C. Hartman. 1987. Adolescent Runaways: Causes and Consequences. Lexington, Mass.: D. C. Heath, Lexington Books.

Kronenfeld, D., M. Phillips, and V. Middleton-Jeter. 1980. The forgotten ones: Treatment of single parent multi-problem families in a residential setting. Prepared under Grant no. 18-P-90705/03. Washington, D.C.: U.S. Department of Health and Human Services, Office of Human Development Services.

McChesney, K. Y. 1986. New findings on homeless families. Family Professional 1(2).

Morse, G. A. 1986. A Contemporary Assessment of Urban Homelessness: Implications for Social Change. St. Louis: Center for Metropolitan Studies, University of Missouri-St. Louis.

Morse, G. A., N. M. Shields, C. R. Hanneke, R. J. Calsyn, G. K. Burger, and B. Nelson. 1985. Homeless People in St. Louis: A Mental Health Program Evaluation, Field Study and Followup Investigation. Jefferson City, Mo.: State Department of Mental Health.

Mowbray, C. V., S. Johnson, A. Solarz, and C. J. Combs. 1985. Mental Health and Homelessness in Detroit: A Research Study. Lansing: Michigan Department of Mental Health.

Multnomah County, Oregon, Department of Human Services. 1984. The Homeless Poor. Multnomah County, Oreg.: Social Services Division, Department of Human Services.

Multnomah County, Oregon, Department of Human Services. 1985. Homeless Women. Multnomah County, Oreg.: Social Services Division, Department of Human Services.

New York Times. October 16, 1987. New Reagan policy to cut benefits for the aged blind and disabled. A1.

Robertson, M. J. 1987. Homeless veterans: An emerging problem. Pp. 64–81 in The Homeless in Contemporary Society, R. D. Bingham, R. E. Green, and S. B. White, eds. Newberry, Calif.: Sage Publications.

Robertson, M. J., R. H. Ropers, and R. Boyer. 1985. The Homeless of Los Angeles County: An Empirical Evaluation. Basic Shelter Research Program, Document no. 4. Los Angeles: Psychiatric Epidemiology Program, School of Public Health, University of California, Los Angeles.

Rosenheck, R., P. Gallup, C. Leda, P. Leaf, R. Milstein, I. Voynick, P. Errera, L. Lehman, G. Koerber, and R. Murphy. 1987. Progress Report on the Veterans Administration Program for Homeless Chronically Mentally Ill Veterans. Washington, D.C.: Veterans Administration.

Rosnow, M. J., T. Shaw, and C. S. Concord. 1985. Listening to the Homeless: A Study of Homeless Mentally Ill Persons in Milwaukee. Prepared by Human Services Triangle, Inc. Madison: Wisconsin Office of Mental Health.

Rossi, P. H., G. A. Fisher, and G. Willis. 1986. The Condition of the Homeless in Chicago. A report prepared by the Social and Demographic Research Institute, University of Massachusetts at Amherst, and the National Opinion Research Center, University of Chicago.

Roth, D., G. J. Bean, Jr., N. Lust, and T. Saveanu. 1985. Homelessness in Ohio: A Study of People in Need. Columbus: Office of Program Evaluation and Research, Ohio Department of Mental Health.

Ryback, R., and E. L. Bassuk. 1986. Homeless Battered Women and Their Shelter Network. Pp. 55–61 in The Mental Health Needs of Homeless Persons, E. L. Bassuk, ed. San Francisco: Jossey-Bass.

Schutt, R. K. 1985. Boston's Homeless: Their Backgrounds, Problems, and Needs. Boston: University of Massachusetts.

Shaffer, D., and C. L. M. Caton. 1984. Runaway and Homeless Youth in New York City: A Report to the Ittleson Foundation. New York: The Ittleson Foundation.

Simpson, J. H., M. Kilduff, and C. D. Blewett. 1984. Struggling to Survive in a Welfare Hotel. New York: New York City Department for Services to Families and Individuals.

Solarz, A., and C. Mowbray. 1985. An examination of physical and mental health problems of the homeless. Paper presented at the annual meeting of the American Public Health Association, Washington, D.C.

Stevens, A. O., L. Brown, P. Colson, and K. Singer. 1983. When You Don't Have Anything: A Street Survey of Homeless People in Chicago. Chicago: Chicago Coalition for the Homeless.

Swords to Plowshares. 1986. Transitional Housing Program for Veterans: A Proposal. San Francisco: Swords to Plowshares.

Towber, R. I. 1986a. A One-Day "Snapshot" of Homeless Families at the Forbell Street

Shelter and Martinique Hotel. New York: Human Resources Administration of the City of New York.

Towber, R. I. 1986b. Characteristics and Housing Histories of Families Seeking Shelter from HRA. New York: Human Resources Administration of the City of New York.

Traveler's Aid Program and Child Welfare League. 1987. Study of Homeless Children and Families: Preliminary Findings. Conducted by P. L. Maza and J. A. Hall.

Tucker, W. 1987. Where do the homeless come from? National Review 39(18):32.

U.S. Bureau of the Census. 1963. 1960 Census of Population. Volume One: Characteristics of the Population, Chapter B: General Population Charactersitics; Part XV: Illinois. Washington, D.C.: U.S. Government Printing Office.

U.S. Bureau of the Census. 1980. 1980 Census of Population. Volume One: Characteristics of the Population, Chapter B: General Population Characteristics; Table 15, Persons by Race. Washington, D.C.: U.S. Government Printing Office.

U.S. Conference of Mayors. 1986. The Continued Growth of Hunger, Homelessness and Poverty in America's Cities: 1986. A 25-City Survey. Washington, D.C.: U.S. Conference of Mayors.

U.S. Conference of Mayors. 1987. Status Report on Homeless Families in America's Cities: A 29-City Survey. Washington, D.C.: U.S. Conference of Mayors.

U.S. Congress, House. 1987. Stewart B. McKinney Homeless Assistance Act, Conference Report to accompany H.R. 558. 100th Cong., 1st sess.

U.S. Department of Housing and Urban Development. 1984. A Report to the Secretary on the Homeless and Emergency Shelters. Washington, D.C.: U.S. Department of Housing and Urban Development.

Vermont Department of Human Services. 1985. Homelessness in Vermont. Montpelier: Vermont Department of Human Services.

Washington Post. September 27, 1987. Homeless in the suburbs: They are different from the street people. D8.

Wright, J. D. 1987. Special Topics in the Health Status of America's Homeless. Special report prepared for the Institute of Medicine by the Social and Demographic Research Institute, University of Massachusetts, Amherst.

Wright, J. D., and E. Weber. 1987. Homelessness and Health. New York: McGraw-Hill.

Wright, J. D., E. Weber-Burdin, J. W. Knight, and J. A. Lam. 1987. The National Health Care for the Homeless Program: The First Year. Report prepared by the Social and Demographic Research Institute, University of Massachusetts, Amherst.

2 Dynamics of Homelessness

INTRODUCTION

As the committee reviewed descriptions and discussions of the causes of homelessness, two rather different concepts emerged. The first emphasizes homelessness as the result of the failures in the support and service systems for income maintenance, employment, corrections, child welfare, foster care, and care of mental illness and other types of disabilities. Homeless people, in this view, are people with the problems that these systems were designed to help. The increasing extent of homelessness can be seen as evidence that these systems are ineffective for various reasons—perhaps because of inadequate funding, excessive demand, or the intrinsic difficulties of responding to certain groups with special needs.

An alternative formulation emphasizes economic factors in the homeless person's lack of a regular place to live. As the supply of decent housing diminishes, more and more people are at risk of becoming homeless. The tighter the housing market, the greater the amount of economic and personal resources one must have to remain secure.

When the need for low-income housing exceeds the available supply, the question is: "Who gets left out?" Some seem to imply that homelessness is largely a random phenomenon for those with the lowest incomes. Others, however, focus on a person's internal and external resources, arguing that when the housing supply is inadequate, those individuals and families with the least capacity to cope—because they suffer from various disabilities, have the fewest supports, or are incapable of dealing with some of the rigors or exigencies of life—will be the ones left out.

Each of these explanations is only partially accurate. Homelessness is a complicated phenomenon, in which the characteristics of local human services systems, public policies, and individuals all play important parts.

PATTERNS OF HOMELESSNESS

Homelessness does not take on a single form or shape. The ways in which housing markets, employment, income, public benefit programs, and deinstitutionalization interact to produce and perpetuate homelessness are complex and vary with the individual. The demographic factors described in Chapter 1 and the personal factors described in Chapter 3 are also important. For purposes of illustration as well as analysis of social service issues, however, it may be useful to categorize various patterns of homelessness: the temporarily, episodically, and chronically homeless.

Temporary homelessness arises when people are displaced from their usual dwellings by natural or man-made calamities, such as fires. A family displaced by a fire or eviction subsisting on a marginal income from part-time employment may be rehoused relatively quickly if local employment and housing conditions are favorable. A regularly employed individual living in a single room occupancy (SRO) hotel or rental apartment who is laid off may rapidly run out of rent money and become temporarily homeless. Once a person becomes even temporarily homeless, reintegration into the community is difficult and may become compounded by secondary factors (e.g., loss of tools, cars, or other prerequisites to finding employment; family breakup; reactive depression; or substance abuse).

Episodically homeless people are those who frequently go in and out of homelessness. A recipient of monthly disability payments or other cash assistance who pays for housing on a weekly basis may be out of funds 2 or 3 weeks into the month. Another example is the chronically mentally ill young adult who lives with family members, but whose situation episodically becomes intolerable and who ends up on the street. A similar situation can develop with runaway and throwaway youths; several studies (Shaffer and Caton, 1984; Greater Boston Adolescent Emergency Network, 1985; Janus et al., 1987) indicate that adolescent running away is not an event but a process involving numerous running away incidents, often precipitated by physical abuse. Both spousal and child abuse also play a frequent role as a precipitant of homelessness for families (Ryback and Bassuk, 1986; Bassuk et al., 1986; Bassuk and Rubin, 1987). Individuals or families, with the latter usually composed of mothers and young children, may double up serially with several relatives or friends but experience episodes of homelessness in between;

they are among the "hidden homeless" during periods when they are temporarily domiciled in other households.

In a Los Angeles study, 15 percent of homeless people interviewed had spent more than a year on the streets without any intervening periods of residential stability (Farr et al., 1986). One-quarter of those interviewed in a Chicago survey had been homeless for 2 years or more (Rossi et al., 1986). These people might be described as chronically homeless. They are more likely to suffer from mental illness or substance abuse than are those who are temporarily or episodically homeless (Arce et al., 1983). However, only rarely do even chronically homeless people remain homeless indefinitely (see Table 2-1); their state of homelessness typically is interrupted by brief domiciliary arrangements, including institutionalization.

Any attempt to estimate the relative proportions of these three patterns of homelessness is complicated by the fact that homelessness itself is a dynamic phenomenon. Many people live perilously at the socioeconomic

TABLE 2-1   Chronically Homeless Individuals (current length of homelessness)

City or State (Source)	Period of Homelessness (years)	Chronically Homeless as Percentage of Homeless Population Total
Los Angeles (Farr et al., 1986)	≥ 1	15
St. Louis (Morse et al., 1985)	≥ 2	16
Ohio (Roth et al., 1985)	≥ 1	21.8
Los Angeles (Robertson et al., 1985)	≥ 1	22
Phoenix (Brown et al., 1983)	≥ 1	27
Milwaukee (Rosnow et al., 1985)	≥ 1	28
Chicago (Stevens et al., 1983)	≥ 1	28
Portland (Multnomah County, Oregon, 1985)[a]	≥ 1	41
New York City (Hoffman et al., 1982)[b]	≥ 1	57

[a]Women only.
[b]Men only.

margin and are at high risk of becoming homeless. A clear and rigid boundary does not exist between those who can fend for themselves and those who cannot; there is a large gray area occupied by millions who are only barely surviving. In the absence of interventions that help to reintegrate people into the community, the proportion of chronically homeless people can be expected to increase over time. On the other hand, intervention strategies that effectively reduce first-time homelessness would reduce the prevalence of chronic homelessness.

Three factors contributing substantially to the recent increase in the numbers of homeless people are the low-income housing shortage, changing economic trends and inadequate income supports, and the deinstitutionalization of mentally ill patients.

HOUSING

There appears to be a direct relationship between the reduced availability of low-cost housing and the increased number of homeless people. Since 1980, the aggregate supply of low-income housing has declined by approximately 2.5 million units. Loss of low-income dwellings can be attributed primarily to the extremely slow rate of replacement of housing resources lost to the normal processes of decay and renewal. Each year, it is estimated that approximately half a million housing units are lost permanently through conversion, abandonment, fire, or demolition; the production of new housing has not kept pace (Hartman, 1986).

From the end of the Great Depression until 1980, the federal government was the primary source of direct subsidies for the construction and maintenance of low-income housing. Since 1980, federal support for subsidized housing has been reduced by 60 percent, and most of the remaining funds reflect subsidy commitments undertaken before 1980. Federal support for development of new low-income housing has essentially disappeared (U.S. Congress, House, Committee on Ways and Means, 1987). Concurrently, there has been a failure to replace SRO housing lost to conversion, gentrification, and urban renewal. In many cities, SRO housing has been the primary source of housing for the elderly poor, for seasonally employed single workers, and for chronically disabled people (Hope and Young, 1984, 1986; Hopper and Hamberg, 1984). Since 1970, 1 million SRO units—half the national total—have been lost to conversion or demolition (Mapes, 1985). For example, in New York City, from January 1975 to April 1981, the number of SRO units and low-cost hotel rooms fell from 50,454 to 18,853; the SRO unit vacancy rate dropped from 26 percent to less than 1 percent (Mair, 1986). In Chicago during the relatively short period from 1980 to 1983, SRO unit capacity declined by almost one-fourth (Rossi et al., 1986).

With less low-income housing to go around, the relative price of the remaining units has risen dramatically and with it the percentage of people who must pay a disproportionate share of their income for housing costs. Thirty percent of one's income is generally viewed by economists as the maximum one should pay for housing. But, according to the U.S. General Accounting Office (1985), the proportion of low-income renters paying 70 percent or more of their income for housing has risen from 21 percent in 1975 to 30 percent in 1983. The 1983 Housing Census reported that 7 million households lived in "overcrowded" conditions (more than one person per room); 700,000 lived in conditions described as "extremely overcrowded" (1.5 people per room). Almost 10 percent of all households with annual incomes of between $3,000 and $7,000 lived in overcrowded units (Dolbeare, 1983; Hartman, 1986).

Overcrowded housing is directly related to the phenomenon of homelessness. In a typical situation, two or more families are doubled up in a housing unit that should only accommodate one family. For example, the New York City Housing Authority, relying primarily on readings of water usage, estimated in 1983 that some 17,000 families were illegally doubled up in its 150,000 units and described the problem as growing geometrically (Rule, 1983). The stresses produced by that arrangement, including tensions in relationships among the various people who are living together, often lead to displacement of individuals, families, or both. These people may double up again, turn to the shelters, or find themselves on the streets.

The nature of the housing market varies dramatically from one community to another. For example, in the committee's site visits, the shortage of low-income housing for families was repeatedly cited as the single greatest cause of family homelessness in most cities, but service providers in Milwaukee reported an adequate supply of housing for families receiving Aid to Families with Dependent Children (AFDC). In Chicago, the loss of SRO units was perceived as being much more important, although concern was also expressed for the quality of family housing. The committee concluded that despite the regional variation, the lack of decent, affordable housing is a major reason why so many people are homeless in the United States.

INCOME AND EMPLOYMENT

Broad-based economic trends have also contributed to the growing numbers of homeless people. In the two decades between 1966 and 1985, the number of people in poverty in the United States rose from a low of 23 million in 1973 to a high of 34 million in 1984, declining slightly to 33 million in 1985, the last year for which figures have been published.

Concurrently, the composition of the poor population is changing: The proportion of the poor who are aged is declining, but nonaged adults and individuals living in female-headed families are both increasing (U.S. Congress, House, Committee on Ways and Means, 1987).

At the same time, there have been major shifts in the labor market. Total unemployment peaked at 10.7 percent in 1982 (Sebastian, 1985), but a decreasing demand for casual and low-skilled labor has kept the unemployment rate at or near 6–7 percent. Unemployment among minority men has remained at historically high levels (U.S. Bureau of the Census, 1986), and although the gap in wages between men and women has lessened, it still remains. This latter factor has specifically affected families headed by women. In addition, the national minimum wage has not been raised since 1981, even in the face of inflation. These factors have contributed to the recent emergence of a large group of working homeless.

While the number of poor and unemployed people has increased, the availability and the real value of publicly financed benefits has declined. Because of the changes in the character of unemployment, fewer of the unemployed actually receive unemployment compensation benefits. Current estimates are that only one-third of the unemployed are eligible for such benefits. Welfare programs, such as AFDC and state-operated general assistance programs for single adults and two-parent families, have not kept pace with inflation. In terms of eligibility and enrollment, they have not kept up with the increased needs. Nationwide, between 1970 and 1985, median AFDC benefits declined by about one-third in real dollars; in only 3 of the 50 states do such benefits exceed the poverty level (U.S. Congress, House, Committee on Ways and Means, 1987). Similarly, for adult individuals during the 1970s, the real value of general assistance benefits, in states that provided them, fell by 32 percent (Hopper and Hamberg, 1984). In Massachusetts, general relief benefits for an adult individual are now $268.90 per month (Flynn, 1986); in Illinois, they are $144 per month. Those amounts, which are intended to cover all living costs, will not pay for even the most minimally adequate SRO housing in Boston or Chicago.

Although these benefits are inadequate, many homeless people do not even receive them: For example, only half of the homeless in Chicago (Rossi et al., 1986) and only one-third in Boston (Flynn, 1986) receive them. Eligibility procedures in many jurisdictions are designed to discourage applications; but even when they are not, documentation requirements and waiting periods prevent or discourage people from applying. The simple requirement of a fixed address has kept many homeless people from applying or being approved for benefits to which they are entitled. State and local initiatives and, more recently, federal legislation in 1986 and 1987 should reduce that problem; but there is as yet no evidence of substantially increased participation rates by homeless people in public assistance programs.

A particularly controversial cash assistance program in relation to homelessness has been the Supplemental Security Income (SSI) program for the disabled and low-income aged adults. SSI had been a major source of income for the mentally disabled and psychiatrically impaired. Between 1981 and 1984, however, because of legislation that was passed in 1980 in order to clarify eligibility on the basis of disability, approximately 200,000 people were dropped from the SSI program. Many of these people were psychiatrically impaired. Approximately 75 percent of those people were subsequently restored to the program, and the relevant federal legislation has been changed again. However, even the current procedures for obtaining and maintaining SSI eligibility based upon psychiatric disability result in many potentially eligible people going without coverage (Bassuk, 1984; Hope and Young, 1984, 1986).

Some people become or remain homeless while they are enmeshed in the bureaucratic difficulties of obtaining and maintaining eligibility for various kinds of public assistance. In addition to the documentation and residency problems mentioned above, concern with budgetary control and the minimization of fraud and abuse in benefit programs has led to more frequent recertification requirements, greater demands for continuing documentation, and a greater willingness on the part of agencies to close cases for administrative reasons. Although benefits are usually restored, homelessness often occurs during the period when benefits are suspended (Dehavenon, 1985).

DEINSTITUTIONALIZATION

Mental Health System

For the most vulnerable among the adult individual homeless or potentially homeless, the barriers to receipt of cash assistance interact with another set of public policy pressures: deinstitutionalization. In the mental health system, this policy has resulted from three factors: (1) discovery and utilization of psychotropic drugs, (2) concern with the civil liberties of individuals confined in state psychiatric institutions, and (3) greater awareness of the dehumanizing aspects of institutional environments. As a policy, it has been supported and encouraged by federal and local governments, and has led to the reduction of populations in public mental hospitals from a high of 559,000 in 1955 to a low of 130,000 in 1980. It has also been blamed for the large numbers of mentally ill people on the streets of major cities in the 1980s.

To what extent are the actions of the reforms of the mid-1960s actually responsible for the plight of homeless mentally ill people today? The American Psychiatric Association addressed this issue in a special task force report (Lamb, 1984): "Problems such as homelessness are not the result of deinstitutionalization per se but rather of the way deinstitutionalization has been implemented." The term *deinstitutionalization* refers to two interactive and parallel processes. The first involves the transfer of care for individual patients from an institutional setting to the community; the second involves the development of systems within the community that can provide the necessary array of services—most important, housing—and treatment, care, protection, and rehabilitation of seriously mentally ill people (U.S. Department of Health and Human Services, 1981).

As part of the movement to develop supportive service systems within the community and to avoid the ill effects of institutionalization, a philosophy evolved to reduce dramatically the number of inpatient days and, whenever possible, to avoid hospitalization altogether. As a result, a new group of chronically mentally ill adults has matured who, as a result of increasingly restrictive admission policies, have never been inside a psychiatric hospital. Additionally, for those adults who wish to admit themselves voluntarily into public psychiatric hospitals or psychiatric units of acute-care hospitals, the resources are often unavailable. Finally, for those patients with mental illnesses severe enough to warrant involuntary commitment or for those who are voluntarily admitted, the rehabilitative value of extremely short hospital stays has been questioned. Despite all these problems, however, most patients can be maintained in the community if an adequate range of less restrictive alternatives is available.

Deinstitutionalization and noninstitutionalization have become increasingly difficult to implement successfully because they depend heavily on the availability of housing and supportive community services. In reality, few communities have established adequate networks of services for the deinstitutionalized mentally ill. Various specialized community facilities may be necessary to treat some individuals. This includes, for example, the "young adult chronic" patient, whose mental pathology, combined with a reluctance to acknowledge the illnesses and an aversion to a regular medication schedule, present serious obstacles to effective treatment (Pepper and Ryglewicz, 1984).

There is general agreement that deinstitutionalization has contributed to the homelessness situation in the 1980s (Lamb, 1984). The committee learned of many individual instances in which patients had been discharged from hospitals with inadequate or nonexistent plans for community care. Other cases were encountered in which there were no community mental health agencies to provide housing and necessary support or assistance to mentally disabled individuals. Service providers across the country expressed dissatisfaction with the extent of community-based mental health services.

A critical point in the treatment of a person with a severe mental illness occurs at the time of discharge from a hospital. Extremely careful planning and coordination are necessary to ensure a smooth transition to outpatient care and community living; it is essential that there is an appropriate residence to receive the person. Some people have become homeless either because discharge planning has been inadequate or because plans that seemed adequate at the time of discharge broke down weeks or months later. In some cases patients have been discharged directly to the streets with no particular destination. In the past, large numbers of patients were discharged to SRO hotels or cheap apartments. A discharge plan of this sort seemed to afford a minimally adequate level of community-based housing, and in these situations many patients were able to manage some sort of tenuous adjustment. When the demand for housing in cities led to the destruction or redevelopment of low-cost accommodations, the mentally ill were least able to find alternatives and were at a particularly high risk of homelessness.

Once a person ceases to have a fixed address, the community mental health service system is least effective in providing treatment, maintenance, and rehabilitation services. Thus, mentally ill people who have been discharged to the streets or who have been displaced from a housing situation are less likely to continue to receive the necessary array of services.

As described more fully in Chapter 3, studies of homeless adult individuals in cities such as Los Angeles, New York, St. Louis, Philadelphia, and Boston report that approximately one-third of the homeless people interviewed suffer from a major mental illness (e.g., schizophrenia or severe depression). Such findings do not indicate that all these people would have been considered appropriate for long-term hospitalization, even before the era of deinstitutionalization. However, psychiatric evaluations of a selected group of homeless people in Philadelphia suggested that a substantial proportion of those interviewed would meet current criteria for involuntary hospitalization (Arce et al., 1983).

Appropriate housing arrangements are essential for the successful maintenance in the community of a person with a disabling mental disorder. The prevailing professional view appears to be that a service system must include a range of relatively small residential facilities graduated according to the severity of the patients' problems and the extent of care and supervision needed, up to and including 24-hour-per-day support. In every community visited by the committee, this need was felt, and service providers reported that there was a greater demand than could be met by existing facilities. For example, the state of Maryland, in its *Five-Year Plan for Deinstitutionalization* (Maryland Department of Health and Mental Hygiene, 1984), published a conservative estimate of a statewide need for 3,000 beds in community-based facilities and for 6,500 beds if projections were based on data from other states; current bed capacity in community-based residences in Maryland is approximately 1,000. In neighboring Washington, D.C., as a result of the recent transfer of control of St. Elizabeth's Psychiatric Hospital from the federal government to the municipal government, the District government will need 47 additional group homes over the ensuing 4 years for a total of 1,750 beds. Additionally, the District must establish and accommodate the court-ordered closing of an institution for the mentally retarded (133 homes), the court-ordered closing of a juvenile facility (10 homes), and the reduction of crowding at a correctional facility (214 new beds) (Washington Post, September 25, 1987).

Other Systems

Deinstitutionalization is not a policy limited to the mental health system. The general policy has come to be applied to many institutional settings. Many homeless individuals, particularly single young men, have histories of encounters with the criminal justice system. Many returned to the community without adequate housing or realistic hopes for reasonable incomes. More disheartening are the cases of adolescents and postadolescents who grow out of foster care or child mental health and mental retardation facilities because they are no longer eligible for residentially based services for their age group, yet they have nowhere to live.

Some homeless people have been discharged directly from general acute-care hospitals to inadequate living arrangements after they leave the hospital. The most dramatic of such cases encountered by the committee involved people with AIDS (acquired immune deficiency syndrome) who, as a result of their illness, lost both housing and employment. In the only published report about homeless people with AIDS,* the Institute of Public Services Performance, Inc. (IPSP, 1986) reported that among the 377 people with AIDS in metropolitan New York area hospitals, 77 (including 7 pediatric cases) were homeless at the time of the study (June 1985). People with AIDS who were in the hospital and interviewed by IPSP indicated that they were currently living on the

---

* A study of the problem in New York City done by the Institute of Public Services Performance, on contract with the New York State Department of Health.

streets or in a shelter, and 19 percent listed the hospital as their current housing situation. Overall, 57 percent reported that they needed assistance locating permanant housing (IPSP, 1986).

The issues raised in the original movement toward deinstitutionalization of the mentally disabled—for example, the need to transfer treatment from the institutional setting to the community, the need to have *in place* community-based treatment centers, the need to provide assistance (both financial and professional) to those in the community when necessary to prevent inpatient admission or readmission—are the same as those in the current proposals that we deinstitutionalize our correctional, youth services, and hospital systems. The critical element, the one without which any such efforts would appear to be preordained to failure, is that there must also be a place in the community for each person to live. Clearly, the size of the current system of shelters and welfare hotels indicates that such is not the case.

SHELTERING THE HOMELESS

Of those who become homeless, many turn to the nation's growing number of emergency shelter facilities. It appears that the demand for emergency shelter often exceeds the supply; of the 25 cities responding to the 1986 survey by the U.S. Conference of Mayors, 7 reported that people are routinely turned away from existing facilities (U.S. Conference of Mayors, 1986). Advocates for the homeless have asserted that some homeless people were also turned away in many of the remaining 18 cities as well.

Shelters

Shelter facilities are extremely variable, ranging from 1,000-bed converted armories to church basements with a handful of beds. Many are traditional missions operated by religious groups in or near the downtown areas of large cities; others are recently converted public facilities. Whatever the stated formal capacity, most shelters are occupied at or in excess of capacity during peak nights, especially during cold weather.

Although generalizations about shelters must be made with care, most facilities currently operating as shelters for the homeless were not designed or constructed for that purpose and are barely adequate for their current use. Rows of closely spaced cots or bunk beds in a large open room are common; this arrangement permits neither privacy nor any means of securing personal belongings. Being homeless means no regular place to sleep, no security for personal property, and often no assurance of personal safety. In the larger shelters, guests must often be protected from physical assault. In many shelters, sanitary facilities are minimal. In a few states, minimal health and safety standards for shelters are mandated by state regulations (as in New York) or are a condition for receiving public subsidy (as in Massachusetts); in some communities, they have been established by court order (New York City). However, even in those communities, the relentless pressure of increasing demand makes compliance with even minimal standards difficult.

Many shelters were established to provide shelter and sometimes food for only a few days. This was based on the assumption that homelessness resulted from an acute crisis that would be resolved in a short time. Shelters were not originally intended to be broad-based human service systems and are poorly designed to serve that purpose.

Most shelters operate only at night; the most common practice is to require overnight guests to leave by 6 or 7 o'clock in the morning. In theory, such practices deter malingering and return people to the community at a sufficiently early hour to seek daytime employment. However, such a practice also makes it difficult to provide services and exposes unemployed people to various hazards during the day. Hence, many communities have developed "drop in" or day centers where homeless people can safely spend daytime hours and where services for the homeless can be concentrated. Many shelters also limit the number of consecutive nights an individual can remain, reflecting again an ideology of providing temporary assistance but discouraging permanent reliance on such support. For chronically homeless people, however, such policies not only limit their ability to develop relatively more stable patterns of activities of daily living (e.g., developing a personal grooming routine, maintaining the cleanliness of their clothes) but also impede their ability to find employment as a way out of homelessness (homeless people cannot inform a prospective employer where they can be contacted if they do not know where they are going to be).

Some shelters provide a single meal, but for most homeless individuals food is obtained from soup kitchens and other organized food programs. During the last decade, an enormous network of such programs has sprung up across the United States; as with many shelters, most are organized and staffed primarily or exclusively by volunteers. These programs rely on some mix of donations, government surplus commodities, and purchased goods. The quality of the meals is extremely uneven, and many sites provide only certain meals, or operate only on specific days of the week or at certain times during the year.

In most parts of the United States, shelter systems are organized exclusively to serve adult individuals; most are segregated by sex and are not appropriate places for children. Therefore, because many communities lack an adequate supply of emergency housing specifically for families, homeless families frequently must break up in order to obtain shelter. As a result, it is not uncommon for families to place their children in the custody of child welfare authorities. Many other parents avoid shelters and any contact with public agencies for fear that custody of their children will be placed in jeopardy by the parents' temporary inability to provide housing.

Welfare Hotels and Motels

Federal legislation has provided a program of emergency assistance (EA) to families receiving AFDC who are temporarily displaced from their usual living arrangements. EA has become the primary mechanism for financing family shelters in many communities, largely through payments for hotel and motel rooms or similar accommodations. States have had considerable flexibility in their use of EA funds, but EA can only be used for relatively short-term crises and not for permanent housing. Only 28 states have even elected to have EA programs (U.S. Congress, House, Committee on Ways and Means, 1987).

In cities where the housing market for people with low incomes is not hopelessly tight, EA may effectively bridge the transition into permanent living arrangements. However, New York City's welfare hotels and similar facilities in other parts of the country exemplify the limitations of EA. Such hotels and motels were not designed to accommodate large families, nor were they designed to house families with children for extended periods. Most lack facilities for food storage and preparation. Providing nutritional meals to young children without refrigerators, stoves, or cooking utensils is almost impossible, and bottle-feeding young infants is very difficult.

In addition to being inappropriate places to rear children, such forms of temporary housing are extremely costly. For example, in 1986, the Commonwealth of Massachusetts paid between $1,350 and $1,600 per month per family for this type of accommodation; the annual average was calculated at $16,000 per family (Gallagher, 1986). This amount would secure a spacious apartment in some of the better neighborhoods in many American cities.

In addition to shelters and welfare hotels, other forms of shelter have been created. In many cities, churches have opened their doors to homeless people. Many homeless people prefer accommodations in churches over those in large public facilities. Some who refuse (or are turned away from) shelters use cars, tents, or cardboard boxes as temporary shelters. Homeless people have also described constructing rudimentary forms of shelter in public parks, from Fenway Park in Boston to Balboa Park in San Diego. What is common to each of these forms of housing is that none are appropriate as short- or long-term housing.

Extent of the Shelter System

Various conclusions about basic services for the homeless can be drawn. First, in most cities there is no system. Some cities have established coordinating mechanisms to mobilize emergency efforts during periods of cold or otherwise dangerous weather. In fact, the emergency shelter system was founded on the assumption that the clients' needs and the services they required would be transient and intermittent. Indeed, like the growth of the homeless population itself, mechanisms for providing services to the homeless have mushroomed, but they still lag behind the constantly increasing demand. Effective planning has been the exception, and even communication among service providers frequently occurs only at the most rudimentary level (Wright and Weber, 1987).

The magnitude and nature of the problem of homelessness are unprecedented within the memory of most adults, so there are few past experiences that could guide planning efforts by public officials and community agencies. Adequate services must be provided, but without permanently institutionalizing homeless families and individuals through another human service system that inherently provides second-class services. Shelters are inappropriate substitutes for long-term housing, and attempts to respond to immediate needs can deflect energy and resources from longer term initiatives. Moreover, there are inherent dilemmas in the siting of facilities. There is a growing pressure from the business community to reduce the concentration of homeless people in central downtown areas. However, residents of neighborhoods that might be more appropriately residential tend to mobilize quickly and aggressively in opposition to the establishment of facilities for the homeless in their midst. Dispersion far from downtown areas may further isolate the homeless from such basic needs as, for example, transportation and access to health and social services.

Another conclusion that can be made about existing services for the homeless is that a large proportion of those services rely on the efforts of volunteers. The selfless energy of volunteers and the magnitude and spontaneity of their endeavors throughout the nation have been central to the effective functioning of the shelter network. However, there are some drawbacks to the reliance on volunteer staffs. The continuity and reliability of services sometimes suffer. Many volunteers are associated with religious organizations whose values may conflict with some of the service needs of the homeless. Moreover, the presence of volunteer services, even if clearly inadequate in meeting the prevailing needs, may provide public officials with an excuse to avoid their responsibilities and obligations.

One final point must be made about the existing shelter situation. At no point was it determined as a matter of policy that shelters were to be a substitute for other human service systems, such as those for mental health, education, foster care, and skilled nursing care. However, that is what seems to be happening in many parts of the country. As reported in the Greater Boston Adolescent Emergency Network study of Massachusetts shelters for adolescents, these facilities are not used for emergency shelter as much as they are used to address other problems or to fill service gaps. The committee concluded that the shelter system cannot substitute for other systems, nor can it be expected to address problems for which—at least theoretically—other systems have already been established.

SUMMARY

As has been seen in this chapter, the causes of homelessness are many and interrelated: the decline in the number of units of affordable housing, the increases in the number (albeit a declining percentage) of people among the U.S. population who are unemployed, changes in the economy that have reduced employment possibilities for unskilled labor, a tightening of eligibility standards and a reduction in benefit levels for entitlement programs, the change in focus of the mental health system, and a change in emphasis from inpatient to outpatient treatment of both acute and chronic physical illnesses. The shelter "system," was never intended to address either the large numbers of homeless people or the complexities of homelessness in the 1980s. Various short-term emergency shelter approaches, including welfare hotels and motels for families, are inadequate as responses to the long-term changes that have caused this problem to grow so dramatically. As will be seen in Chapter 3, the state of being that is called homelessness is intricately entwined with the aspect of the individual's well-being that is called health. Solutions proposed to remedy one cannot ignore the other.

REFERENCES

Arce, A. A., M. Tadlock, and M. J. Vergare. 1983. A psychiatric profile of street people admitted to an emergency shelter. Hospital and Community Psychiatry 34(9):812–817.

Bassuk, E. L. 1984. The Homelessness Problem. Scientific American 251(1):40–44.

Bassuk, E. L., and L. Rubin. 1987. Homeless children: A neglected population. American Journal of Orthopsychiatry 5(2):1–9.

Bassuk, E. L., L. Rubin, and A. Lauriat. 1984. Is homelessness a mental health problem? American Journal of Psychiatry 141(12):1546–1550.

Bassuk, E. L., L. Rubin, and A. Lauriat. 1986. Characteristics of sheltered homeless families. American Journal of Public Health 76(September):1097–1101.

Brown, C. E., S. MacFarlane, R. Paredes, and L. Stark. 1983. The Homeless of Phoenix: Who Are They and What Should Be Done? Phoenix, Ariz.: Phoenix South Community Mental Health Center.

Dehavenon, A. L. 1985. The tyranny of indifference and the reinstitutionalization of hunger, homelessness, and poor health: A study of the causes and conditions of the food emergency in 1,506 households with children in East Harlem, Brooklyn, and the Bronx in 1984. Paper prepared for the East Harlem Interfaith Welfare Committee. New York: East Harlem Interfaith Welfare Committee.

Dolbeare, C. 1983. The low income housing crisis. In America's Housing Crisis: What Is To Be Done?, C. Hartman, ed. Boston: Routledge and Kegan.

Farr, R. K., P. Koegel, and A. Burnam. 1986. A Study of Homelessness and Mental Illness in the Skid Row Area of Los Angeles. Los Angeles: Los Angeles County Department of Mental Health.

Flynn, R. L. 1986. Making Room: Comprehensive Policy for the Homeless. Boston: City of Boston.

Gallagher, E. 1986. No Place Like Home: A Report on the Tragedy of Homeless Children and Their Families in Massachusetts. Boston: Massachusetts Committee for Children and Youth, Inc.

Greater Boston Adolescent Emergency Network. 1985. Ride a Painted Pony on a Spinning Wheel Ride. Boston: Massachusetts Committee for Children and Youth, Inc.

Hartman, C. 1986. The housing part of the homeless problem. Pp. 71–85 in The Mental Health Needs of Homeless Persons, E. Bassuk, ed. San Francisco: Jossey-Bass.

Hoffman, S. F., D. Wenger, J. Nigro, and R. Rosenfeld. 1982. Who Are the Homeless? A Study of Randomly Selected Men Who Use the New York City Shelters. Albany: New York State Office of Mental Health.

Hope, M., and J. Young. 1984. From back wards to back alleys: Deinstitutionalization and the homeless. Urban and Social Change Review 17(Summer):7–11.

Hope, M., and J. Young. 1986. The politics of displacement: Sinking into homelessness. Pp. 106–112 in Housing the Homeless, J. Erickson and C. Wilhelm, eds. New Brunswick, N.J.: Center for Urban Policy Research, Rutgers, The State University of New Jersey.

Hopper, K., and J. Hamberg. 1984. The Making of America's Homeless: From Skid Row to New Poor, 1945–1984. Working Papers in Social Policy. New York: Community Service Society of New York.

Institute of Public Services Performance. 1986. AIDS Shelter Project: Final Report. New York: Institute of Public Services Performance.

Janus, M.-D., A. McCormack, A. W. Burgess, and C. Hartman. 1987. Adolescent Runaways: Causes and Consequences. Lexington, Mass.: D. C. Heath, Lexington Books.

Lamb, H. R., ed. 1984. The Homeless Mentally Ill. Washington, D.C.: American Psychiatric Association.

Mair, A. 1986. The homeless and the post-industrial city. Political Geography Quarterly 5(October):351–368.

Mapes, L. V. 1985. Faulty food and shelter programs draw charge that nobody's home to homeless. National Journal 9(March):474–476.

Maryland Department of Health and Mental Hygiene. 1984. Five Year Plan for Deinstitutionalization. Baltimore: Department of Health and Mental Hygiene.

Morse, G. A., N. M. Shields, C. R. Hanneke, R. J. Calsyn, G. K. Burger, and B. Nelson. 1985. Homeless People in St. Louis: A Mental Health Program Evaluation, Field Study and Followup Investigation. Jefferson City, Mo.: State Department of Mental Health.

Multnomah County, Oregon, Department of Human Services. 1985. Homeless Women. Multnomah County, Oreg.: Social Services Division, Department of Human Services.

Pepper, B., and H. Ryglewicz. 1984. Advances in Treating the Young Chronic Patient. San Francisco: Jossey-Bass.

Robertson, M. J., R. H. Ropers, and R. Boyer. 1985. The Homeless of Los Angeles County: An Empirical Evaluation. Basic Shelter Research Project, Document no. 4. Los Angeles: Psychiatric Epidemiology Program, School of Public Health, University of California, Los Angeles.

Rosnow, M. J., T. Shaw, and C. S. Concord. 1985. Listening to the Homeless: A Study of Homeless Mentally Ill Persons in Milwaukee. Prepared by Human Services Triangle, Inc. Madison: Wisconsin Office of Mental Health.

Rossi, P. H., G. A. Fisher, and G. Willis. 1986. The Condition of the Homeless in Chicago. A report prepared by the Social and Demographic Research Institute, University of Massachusetts at Amherst, and the National Opinion Research Center, University of Chicago.

Roth, D., G. J. Bean, Jr., N. Lust, and T. Saveanu. 1985. Homelessness in Ohio: A Study of People in Need. Columbus: Office of Program Evaluation and Research, Ohio Department of Mental Health.

Rule, S. 1983. 17,000 Families in public housing double up illegally, city believes. New York Times, April 21, A1.

Ryback, R., and E. L. Bassuk. 1986. Homeless Battered Women and Their Shelter Network. Pp. 55–70 in The Mental Health Needs of Homeless Persons, E. L. Bassuk, ed. San Francisco: Jossey-Bass.

Sebastian, J. G. 1985. Homelessness: A state of vulnerability. Family and Community Health 8(November):11–24.

Shaffer, D., and C. L. M. Caton. 1984. Runaway and Homeless Youth in New York City: A Report to the Ittleson Foundation. New York: The Ittleson Foundation.

Stevens, A. O., L. Brown, P. Colson, and K. Singer. 1983. When You Don't Have Anything: A Street Survey of Homeless People in Chicago. Chicago: Chicago Coalition for the Homeless.

U.S. Bureau of the Census. 1986. Statistical Abstracts of the United States: 1987. Washington, D.C.: U.S. Government Printing Office.

U.S. Conference of Mayors. 1986. The Continued Growth of Hunger, Homelessness and Poverty in America's Cities: 1986. A 25-City Survey. Washington, D.C.: U.S. Conference of Mayors.

U.S. Congress, House, Committee on Ways and Means. 1987. Background material and data on programs within the jurisdiction of the Committee on Ways and Means. 100th Cong., 1st sess., March 6, 1987.

U.S. Department of Health and Human Services. 1981. Towards a National Plan for the Chronically Mentally Ill. Committee on the Mentally Ill. DHHS Publication No. (ADM) 81–1077. Washington, D.C.: U.S. Department of Health and Human Services.

U.S. General Accounting Office. 1985. Homelessness: A Complex Problem and the Federal Response. Washington, D.C.: U.S. General Accounting Office.

Washington Post. September 25, 1987. City seeks affluent areas for group homes. A1.

Wright, J. D., and E. Weber. 1987. Homelessness and Health. New York: McGraw-Hill.

3 Health Problems of Homeless People

Homeless people are at relatively high risk for a broad range of acute and chronic illnesses. Precise data on the prevalence of specific illnesses among homeless people compared with those among nonhomeless people are difficult to obtain, but there is a body of information indicating that homelessness is associated with a number of physical and mental problems. This is evident not only in recent data from the Social and Demographic Research Institute but also in individual published reports in the medical literature. It also was apparent to the committee in its site visits across the country.

TYPES OF INTERACTIONS BETWEEN HEALTH AND HOMELESSNESS

In examining the relationship between homelessness and health, the committee observed that there are three different types of interactions: (1) Some health problems precede and causally contribute to homelessness, (2) others are consequences of homelessness, and (3) homelessness complicates the treatment of many illnesses. Of course, certain diseases and treatments cut across these patterns and may occur in all three categories.

Health Problems That Cause Homelessness

Certain illnesses and health problems are frequent antecedents of homelessness. The most common of these are the major mental illnesses, especially chronic schizophrenia. As mentally ill people's disabilities

39

worsen, their ability to cope with their surroundings—or the ability of those around them to cope with their behavior—becomes severely strained. In the absence of appropriate therapeutic interventions and supportive alternative housing arrangements, many wind up on the streets. Another contemporary example of illness leading to homelessness is AIDS. As the disease progresses and leads to repeated and more serious bouts with opportunistic infections, the individual becomes unable to work and may be unable to afford to continue paying rent. Other health problems contributing to homelessness include alcoholism and drug dependence, disabling conditions that cause a person to become unemployed, or any major illness that results in massive health care expenses.

One type of health problem in this category—about which the committee heard much during several site visits—is accidental injury, especially job-related accidents. Although such programs as Workers' Compensation were designed to prevent economic devastation as a result of workplace casualties, they often fall far short of what is optimal for many reasons, including lack of knowledge of the program by the employee, low levels of benefits under the program, and lack of benefits for "off the books" work and migrant farm labor. A case study illustrates the point:*

Samuel Anderson arrived in New York City in 1985 from his native Oklahoma. He is 24 years old, educated through the 11th grade, and says he left his rural surroundings because there was no opportunity to work, ". . . there was no job with something ahead of it." He feels that his chances will be best in the "biggest town I know of." In New York, he is studying for a graduate equivalency diploma and supports himself as an evening security guard. His wages are enough to pay for a rented room in the borough of Queens. Five months after starting work, he scuffles with intruders and suffers gunshot wounds in his right leg and hand (he is right-handed). Mr. Anderson spends 2 weeks in the hospital after losing four pints of blood through his wounds. A vascular surgeon and a neurosurgeon repair his shattered hand during a 4-hour microsurgical procedure. In the meantime, his room in Queens (he is in a hospital in the borough of Manhattan, some distance away) is rented to someone else because of his absence and the concurrent lack of rent payment. After discharge from the hospital, he spends a few nights in a hotel. When his money runs out, he sleeps in a city park, finally coming to a shelter.

In addition to accidents, various common illnesses such as the degenerative diseases that accompany old age can also lead to homelessness:

---

*Unless otherwise noted, all case studies in this chapter are drawn from a background paper prepared for this report, "Homelessness: A Medical Viewpoint," (Vicic and Doherty, 1987) by William Vicic, M.D., and Patricia Doherty, R.N., of St. Vincent's Hospital Medical Center, New York City. The names, of course, are fictitious; the circumstances and clinical details are real and are drawn from Dr. Vicic's and Ms. Doherty's professional experiences working with the homeless.

James Barnam, now 62 years old, has worked regularly since age 17, but has never found a job with secure employee benefits. He has lived a marginal existence: adequate funds for food and a room in a single room occupancy hotel, but certainly not enough for savings. He is fired from his long-held kitchen job because he cannot see the food stains on the dishes; after working 2 days as a messenger, he is let go because items were delivered to incorrect addresses. Mr. Barnam has eye cataracts, a frequent accompaniment of older age and treatable with ambulatory surgery for those patients with health insurance. Mr. Barnam's marginal income entitles him to Medicaid benefits, but he is unable to negotiate the public welfare system and has no one to guide him through forms, appointments, and examinations. Upon losing his hotel room, Mr. Barnam goes to a shelter for homeless men after he is discovered at a bus station by outreach workers. However, even there, his health problem remains troublesome: he almost loses his bed because he fails to sign a daily bed roster he cannot see.

In each of these cases, employment was not secure, and the man lacked a network of family or friends. The fact that health problems precipitated homelessness underscores the relationships among health status, employment, social supports, and access to affordable housing.

Health Problems That Result from Being Homeless

Homelessness increases the risk of developing health problems such as diseases of the extremities and skin disorders; it increases the possibility of trauma, especially as a result of physical assault or rape (Kelly, 1985).* It can also turn a relatively minor health problem into a serious illness, as can be seen by the case of Doris Foy:

Doris Foy's varicose veins occasionally result in swollen ankles. When homeless, she sleeps upright, and her legs swell so severely that tissue breakdown develops into open lacerations. She covers these with cloth and stockings— enough to absorb the drainage but also to cause her to be repugnant to others because of the smell and unsightly brown stains. She is eventually brought to a clinic by an outreach worker. When the cloth and the stockings are removed from the legs, there are maggots in the wounds. She is taken to the emergency room of a hospital, where her wounds are cleaned.

Other health problems that may result from or that are commonly associated with homelessness include malnutrition, parasitic infestations, dental and periodontal disease, degenerative joint diseases, venereal diseases, hepatic cirrhosis secondary to alcoholism, and infectious hepatitis related to intravenous (IV) drug abuse.

---

*In several site visits, committee members heard repeated reference to the high prevalence of sexual assaults against homeless women. One shelter staff member commented: "It's not a question of whether a homeless woman will be raped, but simply a question of when."

Homelessness as a Complicating Factor in Health Care

For even the most routine medical treatment, the state of being homeless makes the provision of care extraordinarily difficult. Even the need for bed rest is complicated, if not impossible, when the patient does not have a bed or, as is the case in many shelters for the homeless, must leave the shelter in the early morning. Diabetes, for example, usually is not difficult to treat in a domiciled person. For most people, daily insulin injections and control of diet are adequate. In a homeless person, however, treatment is virtually impossible: Some types of insulin need to be refrigerated; syringes may be stolen (in cities where IV drug abuse is common, syringes have a high street value) or, sometimes, the homeless diabetic may be mistaken for an IV drug abuser; and diet cannot be controlled because soup kitchens serve whatever they can get, which rules out special therapeutic diets. The following case illustrates the various problems involved in treating a homeless man with another common chronic medical problem, hypertension:

Tyrone Harrison is black, 26 years old, and homeless because he cannot find a job. He wants to work in the shelter kitchen and waits 3 hours for a preemployment physical examination. He is friendly and describes himself as "very healthy." His blood pressure is 180/120. His smile disappears and he feels "cut down." Because he is homeless, he must deal with his illness, private and asymptomatic, in the public spaces of the shelter. He refuses to talk about high blood pressure with the fellows in the dormitory—it diminishes his macho image. He tells the nurse that his blood pressure reading must be a mistake. Three weeks later, after six contacts with the medical outreach worker, he confides that his cousin had been a dialysis patient because of hypertensive kidney disease. Weeks later, after several more visits to the medical team, Tyrone consents to medication for his persistently elevated blood pressure. His 2-week supply of pills are stolen 4 days later. An argument erupts in the dormitory and, in accord with routine regulations, Tyrone is put out of the shelter for 2 weeks. On his return to the shelter, his blood pressure is uncontrolled because he had no medication.

The cases described above exemplify not only how homelessness complicates treatment but how burdens are placed on various parts of the social system and on the homeless persons themselves. Because he lacked any form of health insurance, Samuel Anderson did not receive rehabilitation therapy for his right hand, and as a result developed stiffness and had significant loss of fine and gross motor skills; he had to apply for permanent disability benefits. Doris Foy was admitted to the hospital, because the treatment for her leg ulcers, which consisted of elevating her leg and taking prescribed antibiotics, is impossible for a homeless patient. Not only does her hospital stay make a bed unavailable for someone else who might possibly be in more serious need of inpatient treatment, but it also means that the hospital will not be reimbursed for her treatment because under the present system of utilization review, cellulitis with leg ulcers is judged to be treatable on an outpatient basis, and therefore, inpatient treatment for this condition may not be covered by Medicaid.

GENERAL HEALTH PROBLEMS OF HOMELESS ADULTS

Although homeless people are susceptible to the same range of diseases that occurs in the general population, the conditions discussed below appear to be especially prevalent among homeless people. Tables 3-1 through 3-6 delineate the prevalence of various acute, chronic, and infectious diseases among homeless people. A section providing a key to the abbreviations and some other explanatory notes follows the text (pp. 69–71). These tables were developed by the Social and Demographic Research Institute (SADRI) of the University of Massachusetts, Amherst, and are based on the reports from 16 of the Johnson-Pew Health Care for the Homeless (HCH) projects during their first year of full operation (Wright et al., 1987b). The prevalence rates are given both for the total number of people seen and for those seen more than once (Tables 3-1, 3-3, and 3-5). This group of tables is divided further by sex, ethnic group, and age (Tables 3-2, 3-4, and 3-6). The comparable prevalence rates for the domiciled general population are available from the National Ambulatory Medical Care Survey (NAMCS) of 1979, a study of a random sample of adult patients' visits to doctors' offices throughout the United States conducted by the U.S. Department of Health and Human Services (1979). It should be noted that the SADRI data are for homeless people who sought health care from facilities available to them; therefore, they may not be truly representative of all homeless people. Because the NAMCS figures are derived from doctors' offices—not hospital emergency rooms, clinics, outpatient departments, and so on—the sample is not weighted for people in the lowest socioeconomic groups. The two data sets also differ in age, gender, and ethnicity (older white women were more commonly involved in the NAMCS data, whereas nonwhite men were more prominent in the SADRI data). Although comparisons between these figures are inexact, they do provide general measures of the severity and frequency of certain medical conditions seen among the homeless as compared with those among the general patient population seen in doctors' offices.

Traumatic Disorders

Contusions, lacerations, sprains, bruises, and superficial burns are more commonly reported in the homeless population (TRAUMA in

TABLE 3-1   Rates of Occurrence (in percent) of Acute Physical
Disorders in the Johnson-Pew HCH Client Population

Diagnosis	All Adults (N = 23,745)	Adults Seen More Than Once				
		Total (N = 11,886)	Men (N = 8,329)	Women (N = 3,468)	White (N = 5,659)	Not White (N = 5,928)
INF	3.3	4.9	4.8	4.8	6.3	3.5
NUTDEF	1.2	1.9	1.7	2.4	2.2	1.6
OBESE	1.5	2.3	1.4	4.5	2.7	2.1
MINURI	23.6	33.2	33.4	32.8	36.0	30.8
SERRI	2.2	3.4	3.9	2.5	3.7	3.3
MINSKIN	9.8	13.9	14.1	13.5	15.7	12.4
SERSKIN	2.7	4.2	4.6	3.4	5.1	3.5
TRAUMA						
ANY	NA	23.4	26.3	16.7	25.2	22.1
FX	3.1	4.5	5.4	2.5	5.2	4.0
SPR	5.1	7.1	7.6	5.9	8.1	6.2
BRU	4.0	5.6	5.7	5.3	6.1	5.2
LAC	6.3	8.6	10.5	4.3	8.9	8.5
ABR	1.5	2.2	2.6	1.3	2.5	1.9
BURN	0.8	1.1	1.2	0.8	1.1	1.0

NOTE: See "Key to Abbreviations and Explanatory Notes," pp. 69–71.
SOURCE: Wright et al. (1987b).

Tables 3-1 and 3-2). Results of a 1983 study indicated that approximately
30 percent of 524 homeless people treated in San Francisco over a 6-
month period presented because of trauma-related injuries (Kelly, 1985).
Homeless people are at high risk for traumatic injuries for a number of
reasons. They are frequently victims of violent crimes such as rape,
assault, and attempted robbery. In addition, primitive living conditions
result in unusual risks; for example, the use of open fires for warmth
predisposes them to potential burns.

Most of the findings in the literature, including those from the national
HCH program, describe inner city homeless people. It is not known
whether these observations can be extrapolated to the homeless people
in rural areas. For example, during visits to rural areas of Alabama and
Mississippi, committee members commented on the relative infrequency
of traumatic disorders.

Disorders of Skin and Blood Vessels

Pustular skin lesions secondary to insect bites and other infestations are common among homeless people (SERSKIN in Tables 3-1 and 3-2). In addition, venous stasis of the lower extremities (i.e., poor circulation because of varicose veins) caused by prolonged periods of sitting or sleeping with the legs down predisposes homeless people to dependent edema (swelling of the feet and legs), cellulitis, and skin ulcerations. Although there is reason to speculate that venous valve incompetence would develop more frequently in homeless patients and lead to chronic phlebitis, data are meager. The term "peripheral vascular disease" (PVD in Tables 3-3 and 3-4) is frequently used to connote venous stasis; there is no clear evidence that arterial vascular disease is more prevalent in this population than in a nonhomeless population. Recurrent dermatitis (MINSKIN in Tables 3-1 and 3-2), which is possibly related to inadequate opportunities to bathe or shower and which is associated with infestations

TABLE **3-2**   Rates of Occurrence (in percent) of Acute Physical Disorders, by Age, in the Johnson-Pew HCH Client Population

	Adults in the Following Age Groups Seen more than Once				
Diagnosis	I (N = 3,766)	II (N = 5,783)	III (N = 1,892)	IV (N = 445)	NAMCS (N = 28,878)
INF	5.0	4.8	4.2	7.0	0.1
NUTDEF	1.7	1.8	2.2	3.1	0.1
OBESE	2.0	2.5	2.6	1.3	2.7
MINURI	34.5	33.5	32.7	19.3	6.7
SERRI	2.8	3.8	3.9	2.5	1.0
MINSKIN	14.8	13.7	13.2	11.2	5.0
SERSKIN	4.4	4.5	3.3	2.7	0.9
TRAUMA					
ANY	23.8	24.4	21.8	15.7	NA
FX	3.9	4.8	5.2	3.4	2.2
SPR	7.3	7.4	6.5	4.0	3.1
BRU	6.1	5.5	5.2	3.6	1.0
LAC	9.0	9.2	7.3	4.0	1.2
ABR	2.3	2.2	1.8	2.5	0.4
BURN	1.2	0.9	1.3	0.9	0.2

NOTE: See "Key to Abbreviations and Explanatory Notes," pp. 69–71.
SOURCE: Wright et al. (1987b).

TABLE 3-3   Rates of Occurrence (in percent) of Chronic Physical Disorders in the Johnson-Pew HCH Client Population

Diagnosis	All Adults (N = 23,745)	Adults Seen more than Once				
		Total (N = 11,886)	Men (N = 8,329)	Women (N = 3,468)	White (N = 5,659)	Not White (N = 5,928)
ANYCHRO	31.0	41.0	42.8	36.8	39.4	43.2
CANC	0.4	0.7	0.7	0.7	1.1	0.3
ENDO	1.4	2.2	1.5	3.8	2.6	1.9
DIAB	1.8	2.4	2.2	2.8	2.3	2.6
ANEMIA	1.3	2.2	1.7	3.5	2.0	2.4
NEURO	5.6	8.3	7.7	9.9	8.8	8.1
SEIZ	2.8	3.6	3.9	2.9	3.4	3.8
EYE	5.0	7.5	7.7	7.2	7.0	8.2
EAR	3.4	5.1	4.7	6.0	6.6	3.7
CARDIAC	4.4	6.6	6.9	5.7	7.4	6.0
HTN	10.4	14.2	15.7	10.8	10.9	17.7
CVA	0.1	0.3	0.3	0.1	0.3	0.2
COPD	3.2	4.7	4.8	4.4	5.9	3.6
GI	9.2	13.9	13.2	15.5	15.9	12.2
TEETH	7.0	9.3	9.7	8.6	9.4	9.5
LIVER	0.9	1.3	1.5	1.0	1.4	1.4
GENURI	4.1	6.6	4.2	12.4	7.2	6.2
MALEGU	1.3	1.9	1.9	0	1.2	1.4
FEMGU	11.3	15.8	0	15.8	13.0	9.2
PREG	9.9	11.4	0	11.4	9.2	10.0
PVD	9.1	13.1	14.0	11.1	14.6	11.8
ARTHR	2.7	4.2	4.1	4.3	4.2	4.3
OTHMS	3.9	6.0	6.3	5.3	6.8	5.4

NOTE: See "Key to Abbreviations and Explanatory Notes," pp. 69–71.
SOURCE: Wright et al. (1987b).

with lice and scabies, is prevalent among the homeless population. This form of dermatitis is frequently confused with bacterial cellulitis, since they both present with red, warm, tender skin lesions. This confusion may lead to inappropriate management. Moreover, homeless people do have an increased frequency of bacterial cellulitis and other pustular skin lesions. Finally, homeless people are at high risk of developing subcutaneous abscesses, but this may be related in part to an increased prevalence of needle-stick infections from drug abuse.

Respiratory Illnesses

Acute nonspecific respiratory diseases (MINURI and SERRI in Tables 3-1 and 3-2) are commonly reported in populations of homeless people in shelters. Living in groups, crowding, environmental stresses, and poor

TABLE 3-4   Rates of Occurrence (in percent) of Chronic Physical Disorders, by Age, in the Johnson-Pew HCH Client Population

Diagnosis	Adults in the Following Age Groups Seen more than Once				
	I (N = 3,766)	II (N = 5,783)	III (N = 1,892)	IV (N = 445)	NAMCS (N = 28,878)
ANYCHRO	25.5	42.6	63.1	57.3	24.9
CANC	0.3	0.7	1.4	1.6	3.5
ENDO	1.9	2.1	2.8	3.4	1.6
DIAB	0.9	2.4	5.1	4.3	2.7
ANEMIA	2.3	2.0	2.5	2.5	0.9
NEURO	7.4	9.1	7.8	8.5	1.8
SEIZ	2.5	4.3	3.9	1.3	0.1
EYE	6.6	7.2	9.8	10.6	5.5
EAR	6.0	4.8	3.9	5.6	1.6
CARDIAC	3.6	6.1	11.6	16.2	6.2
HTN	4.5	15.6	27.6	20.9	8.0
CVA	0	0.2	0.6	0.9	0.7
COPD	2.5	4.2	9.3	9.2	3.2
GI	14.1	13.4	15.3	12.1	5.6
TEETH	10.4	10.3	5.8	2.9	0.3
LIVER	0.9	1.6	1.7	0.4	0.3
GENURI	8.9	5.4	5.5	8.3	2.9
MALEGU	1.6	1.0	1.3	1.5	3.2
FEMGU	13.3	11.3	4.5	1.4	7.3
PREG	18.1	4.8	0	0	0.5
PVD	9.8	13.4	17.4	18.2	0.9
ARTHR	1.4	3.4	10.9	9.7	3.7
OTHMS	5.2	5.9	8.0	6.1	5.8

NOTE: See "Key to Abbreviations and Explanatory Notes," pp. 69–71.

SOURCE: Wright et al. (1987b).

TABLE 3-5   Rates of Occurrence (in percent) of Infectious and Communicable Disorders in the Johnson-Pew Health Care for the Homeless Client Population

Diagnosis	All Adults ($N =$ 23,745)	Adults Seen more than Once				
		Total ($N =$ 11,886)	Men ($N =$ 8,329)	Women ($N =$ 3,468)	White ($N =$ 5,659)	Not White ($N =$ 5,928)
AIDS/ARC	0.1	0.2	0.2	0.1	0.2	0.2
Tuberculosis						
TB	0.3	0.5	0.6	0.2	0.5	0.5
PROTB	2.5	4.5	5.4	2.5	3.5	5.6
ANYTB	2.7	4.9	5.8	2.7	3.9	5.9
Sexually transmitted diseases						
VDUNS	0.4	0.7	0.7	0.7	0.7	0.7
SYPH	0.1	0.2	0.2	0.2	0.1	0.3
GONN	0.5	0.8	0.6	1.3	0.7	0.9
ANYSTD	NA	1.6	1.4	2.0	1.3	1.8
Other						
INFPAR	0.2	0.3	0.4	0.3	0.2	0.5
ANYPH	NA	17.4	18.7	14.3	18.5	16.6

NOTE: See "Key to Abbreviations and Explanatory Notes," pp. 69–71.

SOURCE: Wright et al. (1987b).

nutrition may predispose homeless people to infections of the upper respiratory tract and lungs.

Tuberculosis has become a major health problem among homeless people (TB in Tables 3-5 and 3-6). Characteristically, this has been a disease associated with exposure, poor diet, alcoholism, and other illnesses that can lead to decreased resistance in the host. Substance abusers and the elderly are at high risk for developing tuberculosis. Immigrants from Third World countries also have an increased risk of infection (U.S. Department of Health and Human Services, 1980; Brickner et al., 1985). In a study of tuberculosis among homeless people in New York City in 1980 (Sherman, 1980), based on tuberculin skin test reactivity and subsequent case findings, 191 people were initially screened. Of these, 98 had positive skin tests and 13 had positive sputum cultures for *Mycobacterium tuberculosis*. Forty-four required either prophylaxis or treatment according to recommendations of the American Thoracic Society. Compared with nonhomeless populations, these homeless individuals had a very high frequency of skin test reactivity and positive cultures. Whether homelessness alone led to the high prevalence of tuberculosis or whether multiple other predisposing factors were equally important is not obvious from the results of this single study. However, other studies performed in New York City and Boston between 1982 and 1986 confirm earlier observations and support the findings that homeless people have a greater prevalence of tuberculosis (Glickman, 1984; Centers for Disease Control, 1985; Barry et al., 1986; Brickner et al., 1986; Narde et al., 1986). Because tuberculosis is spread by personal contact, these infections pose a potential public health problem to occupants of shelters and to the general population.

Chronic Diseases

The proportion of adults seen more than once in the HCH clinics who suffer from various chronic illnesses (e.g., hypertension, diabetes, and chronic obstructive pulmonary disease) is high—41 percent—compared with 25 percent in domiciled outpatients described in the NAMCS data (Tables 3-3 and 3-4). The high prevalence of hypertension can be explained partially by age, race, and alcohol consumption; but homelessness makes

TABLE 3-6 Rates of Occurrence (in percent) of Infectious and Communicable Disorders, by Age, in the Johnson-Pew Health Care for the Homeless Client Population

Diagnosis	Adults in the Following Age Groups Seen more than Once:				
	I (N = 3,766)	II (N = 5,783)	III (N = 1,892)	IV (N = 445)	NAMCS (N = 28,878)
AIDS/ARC	0.3	0.2	0.2	0	NA
Tuberculosis					
TB	0.2	0.6	1.0	0.9	0.1
PROTB	3.0	4.5	6.9	7.4	NA
ANYTB	3.1	4.9	7.6	8.3	NA
Sexually transmitted diseases					
VDUNS	1.4	0.4	0.1	0.2	0.6
SYPH	0.2	0.3	0.1	0.4	0.1
GONN	1.7	0.4	0.1	0	0.1
ANYSTD	3.1	1.1	0.3	0.4	NA
Other					
INFPAR	0.6	0.3	0.2	0	0.7
ANYPH	16.8	17.7	17.6	18.7	NA

NOTE: See "Key to Abbreviations and Explanatory Notes," pp. 69–71.

SOURCE: Wright et al. (1987b).

the long-term dietary and pharmacological management of hypertension extremely difficult.

Similarly, compliance with recommended treatment regimens for cardiovascular and renal diseases, as well as metabolic disorders such as diabetes, is notoriously difficult for homeless people. For these reasons, many homeless people are referred to hospitals for inpatient care for the treatment of disorders that in nonhomeless people could be managed on an outpatient basis.

Miscellaneous Health Problems

Foot problems occur with a greater frequency among homeless people. These include superficial fungal infections and calluses, corns, and bunions that are apparently the result of trauma from ill-fitting shoes. Homeless people suffer from many dental problems. Reports of poor oral hygiene, cavities, gingival disease, and extractions with no prosthetic replacements appear to be extremely common among homeless people (TEETH in Tables 3-3 and 3-4). These problems are also common among indigent patients in general who have limited or no access to dental care. Finally, various illnesses associated with increased mortality are related to environmental exposure, such as hypothermia and frostbite or hyperthermia (Olin, 1966; Brickner et al., 1972; Alstrom et al., 1975). These life-threatening problems are especially prevalent among alcoholic homeless people and those who abuse other drugs.

MENTAL ILLNESS, ALCOHOLISM, DRUG ABUSE, AND COMORBIDITY OF HOMELESS ADULTS

Mental Disorders

Many homeless adults suffer from chronic and severe mental illness. The visibility of mentally ill people has led to the creation of a stereotype for the entire homeless population; the earlier stereotype of the homeless alcoholic has been replaced in recent years with that of the mentally ill homeless person (Stark, 1985, 1987). One of the first reports describing the high prevalence of mental illness among the homeless appeared in 1978, when Reich and Segal wrote about the Bowery in New York as a "psychiatric dumping ground." They asserted that large numbers of psychiatric patients were being discharged from the mental hospitals and ending up on the streets, a theme that has since been echoed widely in the media and professional literature.

Not only can homelessness be a consequence of mental illness, but a homeless life may cause and perpetuate emotional problems. To sort out these variables, it is necessary to distinguish among the various categories of psychiatric disorders. The major mental illnesses, principally schizophrenia and the affective disorders (bipolar and major depressive disorders), are unlikely to result from the trauma of homelessness. Rather, they cause a level of disability and impaired social functioning in some people that, in the absence of adequate treatment and support, may lead to homelessness, which will then exacerbate these conditions (Fischer and Breakey, 1986).

Personality disorders are not considered "major" mental illnesses because reality awareness is maintained; nevertheless, these disorders are manifested by a person's long-standing inability to deal with the routine demands of living (e.g., as a parent, worker, or independent citizen). Deeply ingrained maladaptive behavior patterns, which usually begin during childhood or adolescence, interfere with a person's capacity to relate to others, limit a person's potential, and often provoke counterreactions from the environment. Personality disorders should not be seen primarily as a consequence of homelessness. Rather, because they impair a person's ability to cope with the demands of life and the expectations of society, they may contribute to the factors that cause certain people to become homeless.

Other psychiatric illnesses, such as the anxiety and phobic disorders and milder depressive reactions, can either be contributing factors in causing homelessness or, more commonly, result from the stress of homelessness. Becoming homeless is a psychologically traumatic event that commonly is accompanied by symptoms of anxiety and depression, sleeplessness, and loss of appetite. Sometimes, homeless people try to "medicate" these feelings away with alcohol or drugs.

Dementia is a progressive deterioration of mental faculties resulting from degenerative brain disorders, such as Alzheimer's disease; recently, it has been observed among some people with AIDS. It can also be caused by repeated small cerebral hemorrhages or traumas from diseases such as untreated hypertension or uncontrolled epilepsy; it is also a relatively common consequence of chronic alcoholism. Certain types of dementia, therefore, would be expected to occur more commonly in homeless people.

In interpreting research data on the psychiatric disorders suffered by homeless people, distinctions among the different diagnostic categories are important. Crude data, such as a history of psychiatric hospitalization (see Table 3-7), are of limited value in defining the prevalence of psychiatric disorders or in predicting needs for mental health services. Estimates of the prevalence of *current* major mental illness range from 25 to 50 percent of individual homeless adults (Bachrach, 1984). The most frequently reported figure—both in the literature and in the committee's site visits—

TABLE 3-7   Treatment History of Homeless
Mentally Ill

Location (Source)	Percentage with Acknowledged History of Psychiatric Hospitalization[a]
New York City (Streuning, 1986)	11.2
Los Angeles (Farr et al., 1986)	14.8
Phoenix (Brown et al., 1983)	17
Portland (Multnomah County, Oregon, 1985)[b]	18
New York City (Crystal et al., 1982)[c]	33.2
Portland (Multnomah County, Oregon, 1984)	19
Los Angeles (Robertson et al., 1985)	20
Ohio (Roth et al., 1985)	22
Chicago (Rossi et al., 1986)	23
Chicago (Stevens et al., 1983)	23
St. Louis (Morse, 1986)	25
Detroit (Mowbray et al., 1985)	26

[a]By point of contrast, a special analysis of preliminary data from four ECAs performed by the NIMH ECA program at the request of the Institute of Medicine showed that a range of from 3 to 6.6 percent of the general adult population acknowledged a history of psychiatric hospitalization (including alcohol and drug treatment facilities) (National Institute of Mental Health, unpublished data, 1987).
[b]Women only.
[c]Men only.

was approximately one-third. In addition, during those site visits, members of the committee occasionally received reports of homeless people who manifested symptoms that might indicate the presence of mental retardation or other developmental disabilities. However, no studies of this problem could be located, so it is impossible to identify the extent to which mental retardation is present among homeless people.

Some researchers have used screening instruments, such as the Brief Symptom Inventory, the General Health Questionnaire, or the Center for Epidemiological Studies Depression Scale, to measure psychiatric disorders among the homeless. These include studies done in St. Louis (Morse, 1986) and Detroit (Mowbray et al., 1985) and one statewide sample of Ohio (Roth et al., 1985). Invariably, authors who use these instruments report rates of psychological distress in homeless people that are higher than those found in other population groups. These screening instruments provide nonspecific measures of psychological distress and not diagnosis. They are therefore of limited value in describing the nature of mental health problems and predicting the needs of homeless people for services.

Several studies have sought to clinically examine homeless individual adults in shelters (see Table 3-8). Two recent studies reported a high prevalence of substance abuse (alcohol and other drugs) and major psychiatric disorders among this population. Arce et al. (1983) examined homeless people in Philadelphia and diagnosed major mental illness in 40 percent of those studied. When substance abuse, personality disorders, and organic disorders were included among the diagnoses, the figure rose to 78 percent of those studied. Bassuk et al. (1984), in a similar study in Boston, reported major mental illnesses (mania, depression, schizophrenia) among 39 percent of those studied; when substance abuse and personality disorders were included among the diagnoses, the figure rose to 90 percent.

Reports of findings such as these have stimulated strong criticisms in some circles. Some critics object to emphasizing the psychopathology of homeless people as an explanation for their homelessness, noting that failure to provide community-based care and appropriate housing are the crucial factors; they are concerned about "blaming the victim" instead of focusing public attention on the societal problems and political choices that are responsible for the increase in homelessness. Methodological critics point to the lack of standardized clinical diagnostic methods and samples restricted to a single shelter, so that the subjects may not represent the overall homeless population.

One study that addresses both methodological objections is that of Farr et al. (1986), who interviewed a sample of homeless men from various settings in the skid row area of Los Angeles. Trained interviewers, using the diagnostic interview schedule developed for the National Institute of Mental Health (NIMH) (Robins et al., 1984), gathered data on 379 subjects. By this method they determined that at the time of the examination, 60 percent of the homeless men met the criteria for one or more current (within the past 6 months) mental disorders or substance abuse disorders. Of the total sample, 11.5 percent met the diagnostic criteria for schizophrenia, 20 percent met the criteria for major affective disorders, and 3 percent displayed severe cognitive impairment suggestive of dementia; 17 percent met the criteria for antisocial personality disorder, and 31 percent apparently abused alcohol or other drugs. Many respondents met the criteria for the diagnosis of more than one type of serious

TABLE 3-8 Studies on Mental Illness Among the Homeless

Source[a]	N		Percentage with Mental Illnesses in the Following Diagnostic Categories:						
		Schizophrenia	Affective Disorder (major depression; mania)	Personality Disorder	Severe Cognitive Impairment	Other Diagnoses	Primary Substance Abuse Diagnosed	No Mental Disorder Diagnosed	
Whiteley (1955)	100	32	14	19	—	21	14	—	
Meyerson (1956)	101	29	—	61	—	—	—	—	
Goldfarb (1970)	200	33	18	38	—	10	—	—	
Priest (1970)	77	32	5	18	—	9	18	18	
Lodge Patch (1971)	122	15	8	51	—	15	—	11	
Lipton et al. (1983)	90	72	—	11	—	—	9	—	

Arce et al. (1983)	193	35	5	6	—	9	23	15
Bassuk et al. (1984)	78	30	9	21	—	1	29	9
Arce and Vergare (unpublished data)	93	48	5	11	—	12	12	8
Farr et al. (1986)	379	12	20	17	3	16	31	—
Fischer et al. (1986)	51	2	2	12	8	22	31	55
NIMH ECA (Robins, 1988)[b]	274	<1	5	5	<1	—	18	75

[a]For Farr et al. (1986), Fischer et al. (1986), and the NIMH study only, "personality disorder" was defined as "anti-social personality"; definitions in other studies may not be comparable for this column.

[b]Data for nonhomeless men with annual household incomes under $5,000. Data were drawn from random samples of individuals in the ECAs in Baltimore; Durham, N.C., metropolitan area; Los Angeles; and New Haven, Conn., metropolitan area as a special report to the Institute of Medicine by L. Robins (1988).

Primary source: Arce and Vergare (1984).

disorder. When added together, the total percentage of homeless people who apparently suffer from any mental illness or substance abuse problem was 83 percent, a figure similar to those found in the studies by Arce et al. (1983) and Bassuk et al. (1984). Several years earlier, using the same diagnostic method, a randomly selected sample of domiciled people in Los Angeles was surveyed as part of the NIMH Epidemiological Catchment Area (ECA) program (Regier et al., 1984). Farr and colleagues (1986) found that, compared with domiciled men in the catchment area study, homeless people were given a current diagnosis of schizophrenia 38 times more frequently, major affective disorders 4 times more frequently, antisocial personality disorders 13 times more frequently, dementia 3 times more frequently, and substance abuse disorders 3 times more frequently.

A study of men at a mission shelter in Baltimore also used the diagnostic interview schedule (Fischer et al., 1986). As in Los Angeles, data from an ECA program sample of a domiciled population were available for comparison. Disorders in all categories occurred with greater frequencies in the 51 homeless men. Overall, 24 of the men (47 percent) had some current (within 6 months) mental or substance abuse disorder; 4 percent of the total sample suffered from major mental illnesses, and 20 percent suffered from alcohol or drug abuse problems. Using virtually identical standardized diagnostic procedures—but very different sample populations—these two 1986 studies (Farr et al. and Fischer et al.) demonstrated a high overall prevalence of psychiatric disorders in homeless men. It is not clear why the prevalence of specific major mental illnesses (schizophrenia, major affective disorder) was so much lower in the sample of Baltimore mission users compared with that in the sample of homeless people studied in Los Angeles—and elsewhere (Table 3-8). Differences in sampling strategy are the most likely explanation.

Although there is a substantial proportion of women in the homeless population, there are no data on the psychiatric diagnoses of randomly sampled homeless adult women. There is an impression, however, supported by nonspecific indicators of mental health status, that larger proportions of individual homeless women than homeless men are mentally disturbed. Researchers in New York City's shelter system (Crystal and Goldstein, 1984) reported that indicators of psychiatric disorder, such as history of hospitalization or current symptoms, were reported by 37 percent of women but by only 21 percent of men. Similar findings have been reported for homeless people from Milwaukee, Phoenix, and Boston (Brown et. al., 1983; Rosnow et al., 1985; Schutt and Garrett, 1986). Unless a woman has a very severe mental disorder, it is probably easier for her to remain within the family network or, failing that, to find some kind of housing. Therefore, it may be the more dysfunctional, alienated, or disorganized woman who becomes homeless.

Women who are heads of households and who are homeless with their children represent a segment of the homeless population that is growing both in numbers and in proportion. These women have a markedly different psychiatric profile than individual homeless adult women. Bassuk and colleagues (1986) have examined homeless mothers with families in approximately two-thirds of the family shelters in Massachusetts. Substance abuse was relatively rare, but this may be an underestimate since the study was limited to shelters and did not include hotels and motels. Of the mothers, 3 percent were schizophrenic, major affective disorders were found in 10 percent, and personality disorders were diagnosed in 71 percent.* The children manifested considerable emotional and intellectual impairment. The authors stressed that measures to help such families, if they are successful, must attend to these psychiatric issues.

Clinicians who work with homeless people in primary health care clinics confirm the high frequency of psychiatric disorders in their patients. Brickner and coworkers (1985), in listing the common health problems encountered in a primary care program serving homeless people in shelters in New York City, placed alcoholism and then psychiatric disorders at the top of the list. The Health Care for the Homeless program's service data, pooled from sites in major cities across the country, show that, whatever the presenting problem, the primary care practitioners also frequently observed a mental or emotional disorder. The authors estimated that 30 to 40 percent of patients have psychiatric disorders (Wright and Weber, 1987). Clinicians were twice as likely to record a psychiatric diagnosis in white patients than in black or Hispanic patients. There was also a higher prevalence of almost every category of physical illness in patients with psychiatric diagnoses than in those without.

Mental disorders are very frequent in homeless populations generally and among homeless people who seek health care. In both groups mental disorders are found that can be considered both a cause and a consequence of homelessness.

Clinical Problems in Providing Mental Health Care for the Homeless

The central problem for homeless people with mental illnesses is the lack of community-based treatment facilities and adequate housing. In

---

*Bassuk et al. (1986) pointed out that this is "a diagnosis of social dysfunction" and that such a diagnosis might exaggerate the degree of psychopathology in this population. It is best utilized as a measure of functional impairment and as an indication of the extent of the need for help.

addition, the special characteristics of this patient group present particular challenges for treatment. These patients often have already had negative experiences with mental health care, often in understaffed, underfunded institutions, and are determined not to accept further treatment. Some have had unpleasant adverse reactions to antipsychotic medications or remember having been abused in the mental health care system; some homeless people lack insight into the reality of their illness and their need for ongoing treatment, but others who are aware of their problems simply do not believe that they will receive appropriate treatment if they accept an offer of care. In most cases, they lack the support of friends or family, are suspicious of authority figures (including providers of treatment), and are slow to develop a trusting therapeutic relationship. As is the case with the homeless in general, their material resources and access to public support programs are extremely limited (see Chapter 4).

From the perspective of mental health service providers, homeless patients are often perceived as less desirable or less rewarding. They may be slow to accept a therapist's sincere efforts to help, but quick to express their negative feelings about the mental health service system. A therapist may be frustrated by failures of homeless patients to keep appointments; and clinics may be unwelcoming to dirty, disheveled, or disorganized patients who frighten away others.

The treatment and rehabilitation of a severely mentally ill homeless person requires the marshaling of major financial and professional resources. Treatment requires enormous patience; considerable clinical skill; and the capacity to mobilize an array of treatment, residential, and rehabilitation resources to meet the needs of a particular patient (Breakey, 1987).

Although ambulatory treatment for mentally ill patients is preferred in most cases, hospital admission may be necessary for treating some patients with severely distressing and disabling symptoms, or for the protection of others if a person is violent. Psychiatric treatment providers are frequently frustrated in their efforts to help the most severely disturbed because of the lack of access to inpatient treatment facilities. The committee received reports from several cities and states that stated that because the supply of psychiatric beds is limited, some poor patients have great difficulty gaining access to voluntary inpatient care; occasionally there may even be a waiting period of several days at a public hospital for emergency involuntary psychiatric admission.

Consent for outpatient or inpatient treatment often can be obtained from a homeless patient relatively easily. For hospital care, voluntary admission is greatly preferred over involuntary commitment and facilitates the development of a constructive doctor–patient relationship. When a patient is unwilling to accept treatment but is clearly dangerous to him-

or herself or others, civil commitment procedures are available. However, problems arise when a patient is ill and behaves in a manner that is self-jeopardizing or is offensive, embarrassing, or frightening to others. Because these people are not unequivocally dangerous to themselves or others, they cannot be involuntarily committed.

Another problem confronting clinicians is a person who is neither offensive nor dangerous but who is resistant to treatment because of delusions arising from the mental illness itself. Mental health workers may believe that medication and supportive care could substantially help a mentally ill person cope, but the patient is legally entitled to refuse treatment.

Mentally ill homeless people have attracted considerable attention from the news media. One of a series of articles in *The New York Times* in late 1986 called attention to a successful new approach to outreach, treatment, and rehabilitation (Goleman, 1986). The program was described by the journalist as "a partnership between modern psychiatry and older humanitarian traditions." Its various elements—persistent outreach, medication, professionally supervised supportive housing, disability benefits, preparation for employment, and so forth—certainly seem to have helped "Timothy":

A Year on the Road Back

Jan. 23, 1985.   Mental health workers find Timothy huddled in a pile of garbage in a stairwell on West 68th Street. He says the Mafia is after him and laughs oddly. From his confused account, it appears that he has been hiding in garbage for at least two months. He resists efforts to move him to a shelter, preferring the stairwell.

March 4.   After several false starts, Timothy is finally brought into the office of Project Reachout for treatment. One drug, then another is tried. He is put on a regimen of Prolixin, an anti-psychotic drug that diminishes agitation and delusions.

March 11.   Meanwhile, a psychiatrist records improvement in Timothy's mental condition; his thinking is clearer, he is more alert, feeling better about himself. The patient starts to take showers.

March 19.   For the first time, Timothy expresses interest in washing his clothes.

April 10.   He agrees to leave the stairwell behind, accepting a tiny hotel room from the project.

May 19.   He starts working in the kitchen at Fountain House, an organization that helps chronic schizophrenics to take part in society again.

Sept. 10.   After project workers apply in his behalf, he receives his first Government disability payment.

Sept. 25.   He begins work as a messenger at Manufacturers Hanover Trust bank offices. A project worker initially accompanies him to take over if he fails.

Oct. 29. He moves into a room of his own at the St. Francis Residence. There is a cable hookup for the color television he hopes to get. The room is newly painted. On the floor by the closet is a blue plastic bucket containing three pairs of filthy shoes and six umbrellas, mementos of his street days.

Alcoholism and Alcohol Abuse

In whatever setting homeless adults are studied, alcoholism is the most frequent single disorder diagnosed. (The exception is women who are homeless with their families.) Severe and intractable alcohol disorders have historically been thought to be especially prevalent among homeless people. Early accounts often attributed the high frequency of alcohol problems among homeless men to their inherent shiftlessness and failure to obtain gainful employment. Anderson (1923) asserted that "practically all homeless men drink when liquor is available. The only sober moments for many hoboes and tramps are when they are without funds." In 1946, Straus used prevalence figures from the studies that were available then and estimated that, overall, 80 percent of homeless men could be considered alcoholic. More recent studies, however, suggest that this perception may be stereotypical rather than real. It is now estimated that approximately 25 to 40 percent of homeless men suffer from serious alcohol problems, and that this level has been reasonably consistent over time (Mulkern and Spence, 1984; Stark, 1987; Schutt and Garrett, in press). This is nevertheless a high figure when compared with that in the general population, in which the most frequently reported figures are 11 to 15 percent for men and 2 to 4 percent for women. The prevalence of alcoholism for domiciled adults in the epidemiological catchment areas studied by NIMH is 12 percent for men and 2 percent for women (J. E. Helzer, Department of Psychiatry, Washington University School of Medicine, personal communication, 1988).

The emergence of a new homeless population further calls into question the meaning of previous findings. Current descriptive studies reveal a population that is younger and more heterogeneous than skid row populations. It includes (1) higher proportions of women and minority group members, such as blacks and Hispanics; (2) alarming numbers of families with young children; and (3) an increased proportion of people with mental illnesses and histories of drug abuse. Despite these changes, serious alcohol problems are common among homeless adults and remain important in understanding this population (see Table 3-9).

Current studies also document the fact that homeless people with alcohol problems are more often physically disabled than homeless people without such problems. As a consequence, they are more likely to use health care services (Fischer, 1987; Fisher and Breakey, 1987; Koegel

TABLE 3-9 Prevalence of Alcohol Abuse and Alcoholism Among the Homeless (in percent), 1982–1987

Location	Source	Problem	Prevalence
Los Angeles	Robertson et al. (1985)	Problem drinkers	25
Minneapolis	Kroll et al. (1986)	Alcoholic	44
Baltimore[a]	Fischer and Breakey (1987)	Definite alcoholic	49.5
Boston	Massachusetts Association for Mental Health (1983) (1-day census)	Alcoholism	45
Boston	Massachusetts Association for Mental Health (1983) (clinical study)	Alcoholism	29
New York State	New York State Department of Social Services (1984)	Alcoholism	15
Washington, D.C.	Robinson (1985)	Alcohol abuse	35
National[a]	Wright and Weber (1987)	Alcohol abuse	47.4
National[b]	Wright and Weber (1987)	Alcohol abuse	15.5
Los Angeles	Koegel and Burnam (1987a,b)	Alcohol abuse/dependence	62.9
Ohio	Roth and Bean (1986)	Alcohol problem	20.8
San Diego[b]	Wynne (1984)	Drinking problem	32
Portland, Oregon	Multnomah County, Oregon (1984)	Drink daily	35
Phoenix	Brown et al. (1983)	Daily/regularly	22
Phoenix	Brown et al. (1983)	Daily/regulary	26
New York City	Crystal et al. (1982)[a]	Regular users	35

[a]Men only.
[b]Women only.

and Burnam, 1987a,b). Wright and Weber (1987) have identified specific disorders that occur more frequently among homeless alcoholics than other homeless people; these include acute disorders, such as trauma, serious skin problems, and severe upper respiratory infections, along with chronic disorders such as cardiac disease, hypertension, and active tuberculosis.

What is the relationship between homelessness and serious alcohol problems? Observers have indicated that many homeless adult individuals who suffer from alcoholism and alcohol abuse are undomiciled to begin with because of their drinking. In a study of homeless male alcoholics in Baltimore, 59 percent reported that drinking caused them to become homeless (Fischer and Breakey, 1987). Others may have become "environmental alcohol abusers" (Shandler and Shipley, 1987), adapting to a homeless subculture that encourages drinking. For homeless individuals, drinking is often seen as the way to make it through a day (Morgan et al., 1985) or to forget failure (Wiseman, 1987).

In the past, many alcoholics lived in SRO housing. For example, a 1979 study of 2,110 SRO housing residents in New York City indicated that 25 percent were alcoholics (Kasnitz, 1984). With the decline in the number of SRO units nationwide (see Chapter 2), many alcoholic single men and women have become homeless. Today many of the country's emergency shelters will not accept anyone who has been drinking. Instead, many homeless alcohol abusers sleep on the streets.

In sum, the causal relationships between problems with alcohol and homelessness are complex, and precise knowledge of them may not be possible or even as therapeutically relevant as one might hope. There is a large general literature on treating people who have problems with alcohol, even though the scientific evaluation of treatment in this area is relatively recent. Effective approaches to this population might have to include several elements, for example, detoxification, convalescence, and entry into specialized alcohol-free living environments combined with supportive treatment programs.

Detoxification is the indispensable first step in treatment; access to detoxification needs to be widely and readily available. Experience suggests that many people entering detoxification facilities will progress no further, and that a small number of people account for the majority of admissions. It is not always possible, however, to predict who will progress further with treatment; a common clinical experience is that, after multiple short-term admissions, some people elect to continue, and eventually they achieve genuine gains.

In recent years disagreement has arisen over the optimal structure of detoxification programs. Traditionally, detoxification has been undertaken in an inpatient medical setting. More recently, nonmedical detoxification programs have arisen (see, e.g., Annis et al., 1976). The latter have attracted much attention because of their markedly lower cost and reportedly equivalent effectiveness (McGovern, 1983). Ideally, a mixture of both would be available. There is little doubt that many people seeking detoxification can be handled in a nonmedical program (Shaw et al., 1981). However, withdrawal from alcohol in people with serious concurrent medical or psychiatric disorders is best undertaken in a hospital setting; many homeless people fall into this category.

After detoxification, some people are unable or unwilling to take advantage of the currently available rehabilitation alternatives, which at present require entry into a specialized alcohol treatment system. Some of these difficulties could be resolved if there were an intermediate stage in the treatment process between detoxification and specialized treatment (Blumberg et al., 1973; Shandler and Shipley, 1987). The goal of such a convalescent stage would be to facilitate complete recovery from the physical and mental ravages of the individual's last period of alcohol intake. A safe setting, perhaps best outside of, but closely connected to, a medical facility, could provide protection, adequate nutrition, rest, and an opportunity to assess the future realistically. Extended medical and psychiatric evaluations, which are problematic in detoxification settings, could be performed, and consequent therapeutic measures could be proposed.

Specialized treatment and active rehabilitation for alcohol-related problems are complex (a forthcoming Institute of Medicine study will explore this subject in detail). Some homeless people with alcohol-related problems may eventually enroll in specialized treatment. However, access to such specialized treatment is far from universal, and the shortage of facilities is serious. Furthermore, there is an extreme shortage of the specialized housing arrangements that are needed to support rehabilitation efforts. Residential opportunities are essential to enable the alcoholic homeless person to get away from the streets, where inducements to resume drinking are ever present.

Illnesses Associated with Abuse of Drugs Other Than Alcohol

There are few concrete data describing the extent of drug abuse among homeless individuals. Most studies about the homeless combine alcohol and drug abuse together under the heading of substance abuse. Those that separate the two provide some minimal information about illicit drug use. Estimates of homeless individual adults with drug problems range from a low of 10 percent reported by users of Johnson-Pew clinics nationwide (Wright and Weber, 1987) to 33.5 percent for individuals living in shelters and on the streets in Boston (Mulkern and Spence, 1984) (see Table 3-10).

Data from the Johnson-Pew HCH projects in 16 cities show that age, ethnicity, and drug abuse are correlated (Wright, 1987). The strongest correlate of drug abuse is age. As with the general domiciled population, rates of illicit drug abuse are highest among younger HCH clients and fall off with increasing age, especially after the age of 50. This is almost the opposite of alcohol abuse, which is found to be least prevalent among younger homeless people.

One of the problems associated with drug abuse is AIDS and AIDS-related complex (AIDS/ARC in Tables 3-5 and 3-6). Whether this is more commonly encountered among homeless people who abuse drugs compared with the remainder of the drug-abusing population is not clear. Nevertheless, as the clinical syndromes associated with AIDS increase in the general population, especially among those who abuse parenteral drugs, it will be an increasing problem among the homeless as well.

Working from a series of assumptions and data from the 16 cities of the Johnson-Pew HCH projects, Wright and Weber estimated the prevalence of AIDS and AIDS-related complex at about 185 per 100,000 homeless persons in those cities. Meaningful comparisons to the rates of AIDS in each of those urban centers are not available, but one reference point is the rate for the U.S. population as a whole, viz. approximately 144 per 100,000 in 1986 (Wright and Weber, 1987).

Other illnesses more commonly encountered in patients who abuse parenteral drugs are hepatitis, skin infections, abscesses, thrombophle-

TABLE 3-10   Illicit Drug Use Among Homeless Individuals

Location (Source)	Percentage of Illicit Drug Use
United States (HCH) (Wright et al., 1987b)	10.0
Los Angeles (Farr et al., 1986)	10.1
Los Angeles (Robertson et al., 1985)	20.0
Portland (Multnomah County, Oregon, 1985)[a]	17.0
Portland (Multnomah County, Oregon, 1984)	26.0
Phoenix (Brown et al., 1983)	26.0
Boston (Mulkern and Spence, 1984)	33.5

[a]Women only.

bitis, bacterial endocarditis, and tuberculosis. Other, more exotic infections that are not frequent in the United States are more common among drug abusers, such as malaria, which can be transmitted among patients who share needles. SADRI specially analyzed its main data base, which consisted of all clients with two or more visits who abused drugs, and found that some disorders were more common among drug abusers than among non-drug abusers. To some extent, however, the differences could be ascribed to various demographic characteristics, specifically, age and the presence of other disorders such as alcohol abuse or mental illness. Using this series of multivariant analyses, which controlled statistically for age, sex, ethnicity, and family status and for alcohol abuse and mental illness, the following disorders were found more commonly among homeless people who were drug abusers: AIDS, liver disease, cardiac disease, peripheral venous stasis disease, and chronic disorders such as diabetes and diseases of the liver and genitourinary tract. Although the exact relationship between homelessness and drug abuse and these illnesses is unclear, most of the findings are not surprising. AIDS and liver disease, for example, are associated with an increased frequency of hepatitis exposure among drug abusers.

Comorbidity

Finally, a point must be made about the comorbidity caused by mental illness, alcoholism and alcohol abuse, and illicit drug abuse. There is a growing concern among those who work with homeless people about clients with dual and multiple diagnoses (further exacerbated by a higher prevalence of many acute and chronic physical illnesses). For example, the HCH data point to correlations among drug abuse, alcohol abuse, and mental illness. Among drug abusers, 42 percent of the men and 41 percent of the women who visited HCH projects and gave evidence of that diagnosis could also be classified as mentally ill; 59 percent of the male clients and 46 percent of the female clients who abused drugs also evidenced a problem with alcohol (Wright, 1987). In another recent study drawn from a broad geographic base, the Veterans Administration Homeless Chronically Mentally Ill program reported that of the homeless for whom evaluations were performed, 32 percent had combined diagnoses of alcohol and drug abuse. Sixty-four percent had been hospitalized for *any* treatment for mental illness, alcoholism, or drug abuse. Because this latter figure is less than the sum of the prevalence rates for homeless veterans seen for each diagnosis (33 percent reported being hospitalized for psychiatric illness, 44 percent for alcoholism, and 14 percent for drug abuse), it appears that many of these hospitalizations were for dual or multiple diagnoses (Rosenheck et al., 1987).

There are two major problems that relate specifically to homeless people with multiple diagnoses. During the site visits, it was repeatedly emphasized to the committee members by those who work with the homeless that homeless people with dual and multiple diagnoses are among the most difficult to entice into treatment. Second, when outreach efforts are successful, there often are no appropriate programs into which such homeless people can be enrolled. Each separate diagnosis correlates to a specific treatment modality and treatment system. These programs frequently exclude those with secondary and tertiary diagnoses of other illnesses. It is rare to find programs that will address a combination of diagnoses on other than the most episodic of terms.

HEALTH PROBLEMS OF HOMELESS FAMILIES, CHILDREN, AND YOUTHS

Perhaps the most distressing and dramatic health problems caused by homelessness are those experienced by homeless families with children. Although the adult members of homeless families appear to be in better health than homeless single adults, they are still in poorer health than the general population. Using data from the HCH projects in 16 cities, Wright and Weber (1987) described 1,417 adult family members who were seeking health care; they represented 15 percent of the total adult population of the 16 programs. The authors concluded that in comparison with the NAMCS population, "homeless adult family members are . . . much more ill on virtually all indicators than the general ambulatory population." With regard to a specific subpopulation of homeless adults in families, the Coalition for the Homeless (1985) has identified the following problems among homeless pregnant women: lack of prenatal care, poor nutrition, and low birth weight of the infants. In a study comparing homeless women living in New York City welfare hotels with women living in low-income housing projects, Chavkin et al. (1987), using data drawn from birth certificates for single births, determined that pregnant homeless women were more likely not to receive prenatal care, were more likely to have babies of low birth weight, and had higher infant mortality rates. With regard to mental illness, although many homeless mothers have emotional problems, most do not suffer from a major mental illness (e.g., schizophrenia). Furthermore, in contrast to adult homeless individuals, a relatively small percentage of homeless mothers had ever been hospitalized for psychiatric reasons (Bassuk et al., 1986).

Wright and Weber (1987) found that various chronic physical disorders are nearly twice as common among homeless children as among ambulatory children in the general population. Illnesses such as anemia, malnutrition, and refractory asthma were many times more common among homeless children. Acker et al. (1987) concluded that more than 50 percent of homeless children had immunization delays. Although there is no precise information indicating that homeless children are more vulnerable to contracting such illnesses as diphtheria, tetanus, measles, or polio, existing epidemiologic data suggest that they are a high-risk group. Using data from the HCH projects, Wright and Weber (1987) reported that the rate of chronic physical disorders is nearly twice that observed among the children in the NAMCS population in general. Whether geographic mobility and residential instability will make these children a greater health risk to the general population is unknown, but it is a potential public health problem of concern.

While access to food—or, more appropriately, adequate and appropriate nutrition—is a problem for homeless people of all ages, it is an especially critical issue for children and youths. Many welfare hotels where homeless families reside do not provide cooking facilities or refrigerators:

> For a hot meal, families must either violate safety codes by "smuggling" a hot plate into their room or use the little money they have to eat in a restaurant. This means that families usually rely on canned goods, dry cereals and other non-perishable items for nourishment. Lack of refrigeration is particularly problematic for mothers with infants who must devise other methods for keeping milk or formula cold, such as using toilet tanks as coolers. (Gallagher, 1986)

Acker et al. (1987) compared 98 children up to 12 years old who were living in New York City welfare hotels with 253 domiciled poor children who presented at the Bellevue Hospital pediatric outpatient clinics. Homeless children between the ages of 6 months and 2 years were at higher risk for iron deficiency, leading the authors to conclude that "this may indicate the presence of other nutritional deficiencies and should be the subject of further investigation."

In addition to physical health problems, homeless children appear to suffer greater emotional and developmental problems. Kronenfeld and colleagues (1980), in their report on children living at the Urban Family Center, a residential facility for homeless families on public assistance in New York City, found that homeless children were having serious problems in school. Children living in this facility were usually 2 or more years behind their age-appropriate grade level in reading and mathematics, often had discipline problems, and were frequently truant.

Bassuk and colleagues (1986, 1987, 1988) described serious developmental, emotional, and learning problems in a population of homeless children residing in family shelters in Massachusetts. They reported that of the preschoolers tested on the Denver Developmental Screening Test, 47 percent manifested serious developmental delays in at least one of the four areas tested (language skills, gross motor skills, fine motor coordination, and personal/social development). One-third of the children manifested more than two developmental lags. In this study, the school-age children were depressed and anxious; half of them required further psychiatric evaluation. Many had severe learning difficulties: 43 percent had already failed to complete a grade and 25 percent were in special classes. It is difficult to determine the extent to which homelessness per se was the principal variable accounting for each of these findings, but a comparison to poor, domiciled children documented that homelessness makes a major contribution (Bassuk and Rosenberg, 1988).

With regard to homeless youths and adolescents, Wright and Weber (1987) reported that substance abuse, sexually transmitted diseases, and pregnancy were more prevalent among the homeless adolescents seen in the HCH projects than among the same age group in the domiciled population reported in the NAMCS study. The three studies on runaway and throwaway youths discussed in Chapter 1 (Shaffer and Caton, 1984; Greater Boston Adolescent Emergency Network, 1985; Janus et al., 1987), while not specifically examining the general health of this population, reported that the youths that they interviewed were not in poorer health than adolescents in general. However, as with the HCH project population, the major exceptions were pregnancy and sexually transmitted diseases. Both sets of findings might be attributed to the fact that these teenagers tend to be more sexually active at a younger age, even prior to becoming homeless. Given that AIDS is a disease that can be transmitted through sexual contact, the staff of the Larkin Street Youth Center in San Francisco expressed serious concern to the committee members during the site visit to that facility that AIDS may spread among runaway youths.

SUMMARY

Homeless people experience a wide range of illnesses and injuries to an extent that is much greater than that experienced by the population as a whole. First of all, health problems themselves, directly or indirectly, may cause or contribute to a person's becoming or remaining homeless. The leading example is major mental illness, especially schizophrenia, in the absence of treatment facilities and supportive housing arrangements. Second, the condition of homelessness and the exigencies of life of a homeless person may cause and exacerbate a wide range of health problems. Just as ill health can cause homelessness, so can homelessness cause ill health. Examples of this include skin disorders and the sequelae of a traumatic injury. Finally, the state of being homeless makes the treatment and management of most illnesses more difficult even if services are available. Examples of this can be found for alcoholism and nearly any chronic illness, such as diabetes or hypertension. As with all other aspects of the problems of homeless people, data on their health problems and health care needs are partial, fragmentary, and incomplete. Still, enough is known about the health problems of homeless people to provide basic descriptive information and draw inferences for the purposes of programmatic intervention.

KEY TO ABBREVIATIONS AND EXPLANATORY NOTES FOR TABLES 3-1 TO 3-6

The data in the tables indicate the percentage of the various subgroups within the client population who have been diagnosed with the various disorders listed. Thus, in Table 3-1, 23.6 percent of all adult clients ever seen (in 16 cities through the end of June 1986; $N = 23,745$ adult clients) have had a minor upper respiratory infection. Among clients (same cities and time frame) seen more than once ($N = 11,886$), the percentage with a minor upper respiratory infection is 33.2 percent, and so on through the tables. The rates of occurrence are given for adult clients only in 16 cities and are for the total number of people seen and for those seen more than once. This latter group is then divided further by sex, ethnic group, and age. In all tables, "NA" indicates that the data are not available at this time.

In Tables 3-2, 3-4, and 3-6, age groups are as follows: I = 16–29; II = 30–49; III = 50–64; IV = 64+. The last (rightmost) columns of numbers in Tables 3-2, 3-4, and 3-6 show the data for adult respondents in urban areas from the National Ambulatory Medical Care Survey (NAMCS) done in 1979 (U.S. Department of Health and Human Services, 1979).

Explanations or the abbreviations and terms used in Tables 3-1 to 3-6 are as follows:

Acute Disorders (Tables 3-1 and 3-2)

INF	Infestational ailments (e.g., pediculosis, scabies, worms)
NUTDEF	Nutritional deficiencies (e.g., malnutrition, vitamin deficiencies)
OBESE	Obesity
MINURI	Minor upper respiratory infections (common colds and related symptoms)

SERRI	Serious respiratory infections not classified elsewhere (e.g., pneumonia, influenza, pleurisy)
MINSKIN	Minor skin ailments (e.g., sunburn, contact dermatitis, psoriasis, corns, calluses)
SERSKIN	Serious skin disorders (e.g., carbuncles, cellulitis, impetigo, abscesses)
TRAUMA	Injuries
ANY	Any trauma
FX	Fractures
SPR	Sprains and strains
BRU	Bruises, contusions
LAC	Lacerations, wounds
ABR	Superficial abrasions
BURN	Burns of all severity

Chronic Disorders (Tables 3-3 and 3-4)

ANYCHRO	Any chronic physical disorder
CANC	Cancer, any site
ENDO	Endocrinological disorders (e.g., goiter, thyroid, pancreas disease)
DIAB	Diabetes mellitus
ANEMIA	Anemia and related disorders of the blood
NEURO	Neurological disorders, not including seizures (e.g., Parkinson's disease, multiple sclerosis, migraine headaches, neuritis, neuropathies)
SEIZ	Seizure disorders (including epilepsy)
EYE	Disorders of the eyes (e.g., cataracts, glaucoma, decreased vision)
EAR	Disorders of the ears (e.g., otitis, deafness, cerumen impaction)
CARDIAC	Heart and circulatory disorders, not including hypertension and cerebrovascular accidents
HTN	Hypertension
CVA	Cerebrovascular accidents/stroke
COPD	Chronic obstructive pulmonary disease
GI	Gastrointestinal disorders (e.g., ulcers, gastritis, hernias)
TEETH	Dentition problems (predominantly caries)
LIVER	Liver diseases (e.g., cirrhosis, hepatitis, ascites, enlarged liver or spleen)
GENURI	General genitourinary problems common to either sex (e.g., kidney, bladder problems, incontinence)

MALEGU   Genitourinary problems found among men (e.g., penile disorders, testicular dysfunction, male infertility) (Note: Data on MALEGU shown in the table are for *men only* in all cases.)

FEMGU   Genitourinary problems found among women (e.g., ovarian dysfunction, genital prolapse, menstrual disorders)

PREG   Pregnancies (Note: Data on FEMGU and PREG shown in the table are for *women only* in all cases.)

PVD   Peripheral vascular diseases

ARTHR   Arthritis and related problems

OTHMS   All musculoskeletal disorders other than arthritis

Infectious and Communicable Disorders (Tables 3-5 and 3-6)

AIDS/ARC   Acquired immune deficiency syndrome, AIDS-related complex

TB   Active tuberculosis infection, any site

PROTB   Prophylactic anti-TB therapeutic regimen

ANYTB   Either TB or PROTB or both

VDUNS   Unspecified veneral disease, herpes

SYPH   Syphilis

GONN   Gonnorhea

ANYSTD   VDUNS, SYMPH, or GONN, or any combination

INFPAR   Infectious and parasitic diseases (e.g., septicemia, amebiasis, diphtheria, tetanus)

ANYPH   AIDS, ANYTB, ANYSTD, INFPAR, SERURI, INF, or SERSKIN, or any combination of these

REFERENCES

Acker, P. J., A. H. Fierman, and B. P. Dreyer. 1987. An assessment of parameters of health care and nutrition in homeless children. American Journal of Diseases of Children 141(4):388.

Alstrom, C. H., R. Lindelius, and L. Salum. 1975. Mortality among homeless men. British Journal of Addiction 70:245–252.

Anderson, N. 1923. The Hobo, The Sociology of the Homeless Man. Chicago: University of Chicago Press.

Annis, H., N. Geisbrecht, A. Ogborne, and R. B. Smart. 1976. Task Force II Report on the Operation and Effectiveness of the Ontario Detoxification System. Toronto: Addiction Research Foundation of Ontario.

Arce, A. A., and M. J. Vergare. 1984. Identifying and characterizing the mentally ill among the homeless. Pp. 75–89 in The Homeless Mentally Ill, H. R. Lamb, ed. Washington, D.C.: American Psychiatric Association.

Arce, A. A., M. Tadlock, and M. J. Vergare. 1983. A psychiatric profile of street people admitted to an emergency shelter. Hospital and Community Psychiatry 34(9):812–817.

Bachrach, L. L. 1984. The homeless mentally ill and mental health services: An analytical review of the literature. Pp. 11–53 in The Homeless Mentally Ill, H. R. Lamb, ed. Washington, D.C.: American Psychiatric Association.

Barry, M. A., C. Wall, L. Shirley, J. Bernardo, P. Schwingl, E. Brigandi, and G. A. Lamb. 1986. Tuberculosis screening in Boston's homeless shelters. Public Health Reports 101(5):487–494.

Bassuk, E. L., and L. Rosenberg. 1988. Why does family homelessness occur? A case-control study. American Journal of Public Health 78(7):783–788.

Bassuk, E. L., and L. Rubin. 1987. Homeless children: A neglected population. American Journal of Orthopsychiatry 5(2):1–9.

Bassuk, E. L., L. Rubin, and A. Lauriat. 1984. Is homelessness a mental health problem? American Journal of Psychiatry 141(12):1546–1550.

Bassuk, E. L., L. Rubin, and A. Lauriat. 1986. Characteristics of sheltered homeless families. American Journal of Public Health 76(September):1097–1101.

Blumberg, L., T. E. Shipley, and I. W. Shandler. 1973. Skid Row and Its Alternatives: Research and Recommendations from Philadelphia. Philadelphia: Temple University Press.

Breakey, W. J. 1987. Treating the homeless. Alcohol, Health, and Research World 11(3):42–47.

Brickner, P. W., D. Greenbaum, A. Kaufman, F. O'Donnell, J. T. O'Brian, R. Scalice, J. Scandizzo, and T. Sullivan. 1972. A clinic for male derelicts: A welfare hotel project. Annals of Internal Medicine 77:565–569.

Brickner, P. W., L. D. Scharer, B. Conanan, A. Elvy, and M. Savarese, eds. 1985. Health Care of Homeless People. New York: Springer-Verlag.

Brickner, P. W., B. C. Scanlan, B. Conanan, A. Elvy, J. McAdam, L. K. Scharer, and W. J. Vicic. 1986. Homeless persons and health care. Annals of Internal Medicine 104:405–409.

Brown, E. E., S. MacFarlane, R. Paredes, and L. Stark. 1983. The Homeless of Phoenix: A Profile. Phoenix, Ariz.: Phoenix South Community Mental Health Center.

Centers for Disease Control. 1985. Drug resistant tuberculosis among the homeless. Morbidity and Mortality Weekly Report 34:429–431.

Chavkin, W., A. Kristal, C. Seabron, and P. E. Guigli. 1987. The reproductive experience of women living in hotels for the homeless in New York City. New York State Journal of Medicine 87(1):10–13.

Coalition for the Homeless. 1985. A Crying Shame: Official Abuse and Neglect of Homeless Infants. New York: Coalition for the Homeless.

Crystal, S., and M. Goldstein. 1984. The Homeless in New York Shelters. New York: Human Resources Administration of the City of New York.

Crystal, S.M., M. Goldstein, and R. Levitt. 1982. Chronic and Situational Dependency: Long-Term Residents in a Shelter for Men. New York: Human Resources Administration of the City of New York.

Farr, R. K., P. Koegel, and A. Burnam. 1986. A Study of Homelessness and Mental Illness in the Skid Row Area of Los Angeles. Los Angeles: Los Angeles County Department of Mental Health.

Fischer, P. J. 1987. Alcohol Problems Among the Contemporary Homeless Population. Department of Psychiatry and Behavioral Sciences, School of Medicine, The Johns Hopkins University. Paper prepared for the Institute of Medicine, Washington, D.C.

Fischer, P., and W. R. Breakey. 1986. Homelessness and mental health: An overview. International Journal of Mental Health 14(4):6–41.

Fischer, P. W., and W. R. Breakey. 1987. Profile of Baltimore homeless with alcohol problems. Alcohol, Health, and Research World 11(3):36–37.

Fischer, P. J., W. R. Breakey, S. Shapiro, J. C. Anthony, and M. Kramer. 1986. Mental health and social characteristics of the homeless: A survey of mission users. American Journal of Public Health 76(5):519–524.

Gallagher, E. 1986. No Place Like Home: A Report on the Tragedy of Homeless Children and Their Families in Massachusetts. Boston: Massachusetts Committee for Children and Youth, Inc.

Glickman, R. 1984. Tuberculosis screening and treatment of New York City homeless people. Annals of the New York Academy of Sciences 435:19–21.

Goldfarb, C. 1970. Patients nobody wants: Skid row alcoholics. Diseases of the Nervous System 31:274–281.

Goleman, D. 1986. For mentally ill on the street, a new approach shines. New York Times, November 11: C1.

Greater Boston Adolescent Emergency Network. 1985. Ride a Painted Pony on a Spinning Wheel Ride. Boston, Mass.: Massachusetts Committee for Children and Youth, Inc.

Janus, M.-D., A. McCormack, A. W. Burgess, and C. Hartman. 1987. Adolescent Runaways: Causes and Consequences. Lexington, Mass.: D. C. Heath, Lexington Books.

Kasnitz, P. 1984. Gentrification and homelessness: The single room occupant and the inner city revival. Urban and Social Change Review 17(Winter):9–14.

Kelly, J. T. 1985. Trauma: With the Example of San Francisco's Shelter Programs. Pp. 77–91 in Health Care of Homeless People. P. W. Brickner, L. K. Scharer, B. Conanan, A. Elvy, and M. Savarese, eds. New York: Springer-Verlag.

Koegel, P., and M. A. Burnam. 1987a. The Epidemiology of Alcohol Abuse and Dependence Among Homeless Individuals: Findings from the Inner City of Los Angeles. Department of Psychiatry, University of California, Los Angeles.

Koegel, P., and M. A. Burnam. 1987b. Traditional and nontraditional homeless alcoholics. Alcohol, Health, and Research World 11(3):28–35.

Kroll, J., K. Carey, D. Hagedorn, P. F. Dog, and E. Benavide. 1986. A survey of homeless adults in urban emergency shelters. Hospital and Community Psychiatry 37(3):283–286.

Kronenfeld, D., M. Phillips, and V. Middleton-Jeter. 1980. The Forgotten Ones: Treatment of Single Parent Multi-Problem Families in a Residential Setting. Prepared under Grant no. 18-P-90705/03. Washington, D.C.: U.S. Department of Health and Human Services, Office of Human Development Services.

Lipton, F. R., A. Sabatini, and S. E. Katz. 1983. Down and out in the city: The homeless mentally ill. Hospital and Community Psychiatry 34:817–821.

Lodge Patch, I. C. 1971. Homeless men in London: Demographic findings in a lodging house sample. British Journal of Psychiatry 118:313–317.

Massachusetts Association for Mental Health and the United Community Planning Corporation. 1983. Homelessness: Organizing a Community Response. Boston: Massachusetts Association for Mental Health and the United Community Planning Corporation.

McGovern, M. P. 1983. Comparative evaluation of medicinal vs. social treatment of alcohol withdrawal system. Journal of Clinical Psychology 39(September):791–803.

Meyerson, D. J. 1956. The "skid row" problem. New England Journal of Medicine 254:1168–1173.

Morgan, R., E. I. Geffner, E. Kiernan, and S. Cowles. 1985. Alcoholism and the Homeless. Pp. 131–150 in Health Care of Homeless People, P. W. Brickner, L. K. Scharer, B. Conanan, A. Elvy, and M. Savarese, eds. New York: Springer-Verlag.

Morse, G. A. 1986. A Contemporary Assessment of Urban Homelessness: Implications for Social Change. St. Louis: Center for Metropolitan Studies, University of Missouri-St. Louis.

Mowbray, C. V., S. Johnson, A. Solarz, and C. J. Combs. 1985. Mental Health and Homelessness in Detroit: A Research Study. Lansing: Michigan Department of Mental Health.

Mulkern, V., and R. Spence. 1984. Preliminary Results of Homelessness Needs Assessment. Boston: Human Services Research Institute for the Massachusetts Department of Mental Health.

Multnomah County, Oregon, Department of Human Services. 1984. The Homeless Poor. Multnomah County, Oreg.: Social Services Division, Department of Human Services.

Multnomah County, Oregon, Department of Human Services. 1985. Homeless Women. Multnomah County, Oreg.: Social Services Division, Department of Human Services.

Narde, E., B. McInnis, B. Thomas, and S. Weidhass. 1986. Exogenous reinfection with tuberculosis in a shelter for the homeless. New England Journal of Medicine 315(25):1570–1575.

New York State Department of Social Services. 1984. Homelessness in New York State: A Report to the Governor and the Legislature. Albany: New York State Department of Social Services.

Olin, J. S. 1966. "Skid Row" syndrome: A medical profile of the chronic drunkenness offender. Canadian Medical Association Journal 95:205–214.

Priest, R. G. 1970. Homeless men: A USA-UK comparison. Proceedings of the Royal Society of Medicine 63:441–445.

Regier, D. A., J. K. Myers, M. Kramer, L. N. Robins, D. G. Blazer, R. L. Hough, W. W. Eaton, and B. Z. Locke. 1984. The National Institute of Mental Health Epidemiological Catchment Area program: Historical context, major objectives, and study population characteristics. Archives of General Psychiatry 42(10):934–941.

Reich, R., and L. Siegel. 1978. The emergency of the Bowery as a psychiatric dumping ground. Psychiatric Quarterly 50:3.

Robertson, M. J., R. H. Ropers, and R. Boyer. 1985. The Homeless of Los Angeles County: An Empirical Evaluation. Basic Shelter Research Project, Document no. 4. Los Angeles: Psychiatric Epidemiology Program, School of Public Health, University of California, Los Angeles.

Robins, L. N., M. M. Weissman, H. Orvaschel, E. Gruenberg, J. P. Burke, and D. A. Regier. 1984. Lifetime prevalence of specific psychiatric disorders in three sites. Archives of General Psychiatry 42(10):949–958.

Robinson, F. G. 1985. Homeless People in the Nation's Capital. Washington, D.C.: Center for Applied Research and Urban Policy, University of the District of Columbia.

Rosenheck, R., P. Gallup, C. Leda, P. Leaf, R. Milstein, I. Voynick, P. Errera, L. Lehman, G. Koerber, and R. Murphy. 1987. Progress Report on the Veterans Administration Program for Homeless Chronically Mentally Ill Veterans. Washington, D.C.: Veterans Administration.

Rosnow, M. J., T. Shaw, and C. S. Concord. 1985. Listening to the Homeless: A Study of Homeless Mentally Ill Persons in Milwaukee. Prepared by Human Services Triangle, Inc. Madison: Wisconsin Office of Mental Health.

Rossi, P. H., G. A. Fisher, and G. Willis. 1986. The Condition of the Homeless in Chicago. A report prepared by the Social and Demographic Research Institute, University of Massachusetts at Amherst, and the National Opinion Research Center, University of Chicago.

Roth, D., and G. J. Bean. 1986. New perspectives on homelessness: Findings from a statewide epidemiological study. Hospital and Community Psychiatry 37(7):712–719.

Roth, D., G. J. Bean, Jr., N. Lust, and T. Saveanu. 1985. Homelessness in Ohio: A Study of People in Need. Columbus: Office of Program Evaluation and Research, Ohio Department of Mental Health.

Schutt, R. K., and G. R. Garrett. 1986. Homeless in Boston in 1985: The View from Long Island. Boston: University of Massachusetts at Boston.

Schutt, R. K., and G. R. Garrett. In press. The homeless alcoholic: Past and present. In Homelessness: The National Perspective, M. J. Robertson and M. Greenblatt, eds. New York: Plenum Publishing.

Shaffer, D., and C. L. M. Caton. 1984. Runaway and Homeless Youth in New York City: A Report to the Ittleson Foundation. New York: The Ittleson Foundation.

Shandler, I. W., and T. E. Shipley. 1987. New focus for an old problem: Philadelphia's response to homelessness. Alcohol, Health, and Research World 11(3):54–57.

Shaw, J. M., G. S. Kolesar, E. M. Sellers, H. L. Kaplan, and P. Sandor. 1981. Development of optimal treatment tactics for alcohol withdrawal. Journal of Clinical Psychopharmacology 1(November):382–389.

Sherman, M. N. 1980. Tuberculosis in single-room-occupancy hotel residents: A persisting focus of disease. New York Medical Quarterly 1:39–41.

Stark, L. 1985. Strangers in a strange land: The chronically mentally ill homeless. International Journal of Mental Health 14(4):95–111.

Stark, L. 1987. A century of alcohol and homelessness: Demographics and stereotypes. Alcohol, Health, and Research World 11(3):8–13.

Stevens, A. O., L. Brown, P. Colson, and K. Singer. 1983. When You Don't Have Anything: A Street Survey of Homeless People in Chicago. Chicago: Chicago Coalition for the Homeless.

Straus, R. 1946. Alcohol and the homeless man. Quarterly Journal of Studies on Alcohol 7:361–404.

Streuning, E. L. 1986. A Study of Residents of the New York City Shelter System. New York: New York State Psychiatric Institute.

U.S. Department of Health and Human Services. 1979. National Ambulatory Medical Care Survey. Washington, D.C.: U.S. Department of Health and Human Services.

U.S. Department of Health and Human Services. 1980. Tuberculosis Statistics: States and Cities. Publication no. (CDC)82–8249. Atlanta: Centers for Disease Control, U.S. Department of Health and Human Services.

Vicic, W. J., and P. Doherty. 1987. Homelessness: A medical viewpoint. Paper prepared for the Institute of Medicine, Washington, D.C.

Whiteley, J. S. 1955. Down and out in London: Mental illness in lower social groups. Lancet ii:608–610.

Wiseman, J. P. 1987. Studying the problem of alcoholism in today's homeless. Paper presented at the National Institute of Alcohol Abuse and Alcoholism Conference on the Homeless Population with Alcohol Problems, Rockville, Md., March 24–25.

Wright, J. D. 1987. Special Topics in the Health Status of America's Homeless. Special report prepared for the Institute of Medicine by the Social and Demographic Research Institute, University of Massachusetts, Amherst.

Wright, J. D., and E. Weber. 1987. Homelessness and Health. New York: McGraw-Hill.

Wright, J. D., J. W. Knight, E. Weber-Burdin, and J. Lam. 1987a. Ailments and alcohol: Health status among the drinking homeless. Alcohol, Health, and Research World 11(3):22–27.

Wright, J. D., E. Weber-Burdin, J. W. Knight, and J. A. Lam. 1987b. The National Health Care for the Homeless Program: The First Year. Report prepared by the Social and Demographic Research Institute, University of Massachusetts, Amherst.

Wynne, J. 1984. Homeless Women in San Diego: A New Perspective on Poverty and Despair in America's Finest City. San Diego: Alcohol Program, Department of Health Services, County of San Diego.

Access to Health Care Services for Homeless People

4

INTRODUCTION

In a nation abundantly endowed with hospitals, physicians, and advanced health care technology, millions of Americans have difficulty obtaining health care. Problems of access to care especially affect the poor, members of minority groups, and residents of most inner cities and many rural areas. Homeless people often face additional obstacles to receiving health care services.

This chapter reviews factors that directly determine how homeless people do or do not obtain physical and mental health services, first, as a part of the larger population of the poor and then, more specifically, as homeless people. It begins by discussing the following questions:

- Why do poor people use health care services to a lesser extent than non-poor people?
- What are the barriers to health care specifically faced by homeless people?
- What is the role of public and private health insurance and the impact of Medicaid in providing financial access?

The chapter then discusses the role of the traditional system of health care for the indigent (including the National Health Service Corps) and examines its role in filling the gaps resulting from the failure of Medicaid to provide access. The chapter then reviews two specialized health care systems: one to treat mental illness and the other to provide services to veterans.

HEALTH CARE OF THE INDIGENT

A right to health care has never been established in the United States either by statute or case law, but a broad base of public opinion generally appears to support the notion that people should be able to get medical attention when they need it, regardless of economic or social circumstances (New York Times, December 1, 1987). To quote from the 1983 report of the President's Commission for the Study of Ethical Problems in Medicine and Biomedical and Behavioral Research:

The Commission concludes that society has an ethical obligation to ensure equitable access to health care for all. This obligation rests on the special importance of health care: its role in relieving suffering, preventing premature death, restoring functioning, increasing opportunity, providing information about an individual's condition, and giving evidence of mutual empathy and compassion. Furthermore, although life-style and the environment can affect health status, differences in the need for health care are for the most part undeserved and not within the individual's control.

The President's commission also stated that "equitable access to health care requires that all citizens be able to secure an adequate level of care without excessive burdens" and that "efforts to contain rising health costs are important but should not focus on limiting the attainment of equitable access for the least well served portion of the public" (President's Commission for the Study of Ethical Problems in Medicine and Biomedical and Behavioral Research, 1983).

Reality, however, has not matched that aspiration. For example, in 1986, the Robert Wood Johnson Foundation funded a study of a random sample of the general public to determine to what extent people have access to health care in the United States (Robert Wood Johnson Foundation, 1987). Along the lines of a previous study conducted in 1982 (Aday et al., 1984), the surveyors interviewed 10,130 people (adults and adults responding on behalf of their minor children), primarily by telephone contact. A separate sample of 300 households without telephones was interviewed to increase the representative nature of the sample. Eighteen percent of Americans surveyed were unable to identify a usual source of medical care—a question that health services researchers consider a benchmark for access to care. It should be noted that 18 percent of the population is equal to 40 million people. The proportion of the population without a usual source of care had increased two-thirds since the survey conducted in 1982.

A somewhat similar survey, the National Health Interview Survey (NHIS), is conducted on a continuous basis by personnel of the U.S. Bureau of the Census. Reports of data drawn from this survey are published at various times by the National Center for Health Statistics, a division of the Public Health Service of the U.S. Department of Health and Human Services. The method used in this survey—personal interviews based on a random sample of households—is generally considered by statisticians to be more reliable than telephone interviews, especially in obtaining a valid sample of the general population.

Comparisons with the data obtained in the Robert Wood Johnson Foundation survey (1987) must be limited because the NHIS survey does not estimate how many people lack a "usual source of health care." However, both surveys asked the respondents if they had seen a physician at any point in the year prior to the interview. The Johnson survey reported that 33 percent of the respondents answered in the negative (up from 19 percent in the 1982 survey). NHIS reported that 24 percent of the respondents answered in the negative in their survey; this was the same percentage as that in each of the previous 5 years (Kovar, 1987).

There are many reasons why people might not use medical care; the most obvious is that some do not need it. In the aggregate, Americans were probably healthier in 1986 than they were in 1982, and young adults continue to use medical care less frequently than do older people. There are, however, certain circumstances under which the need for medical service is broadly supported both by professional consensus and popular opinion, and in those circumstances the Johnson survey found some disheartening results. Seventeen percent of persons with identified chronic illnesses (e.g., diabetes or heart disease) that require regular medical supervision did not see a physician in the previous year; 20 percent of persons with hypertension had not had their blood pressure checked in a year; and 15 percent of pregnant women did not receive prenatal care during their first trimester.

People in fair or poor health with incomes below 150 percent of the poverty level visited physicians 27 percent less often than did non-poor people in poor or fair health; blacks in fair or poor health had one-third fewer physician visits than did non-Hispanic whites. Poor children saw physicians in 1986 as often as non-poor children did, but poor children were three times as likely to be reported as being in poor or fair health. Poor people were somewhat more likely to be hospitalized in 1986 than non-poor people, but they were substantially more likely to have serious health problems of the sort that ordinarily lead to hospitalization. Controlling for degree of illness, the poor received substantially less hospital care, physicians' services, and dental care than the non-poor (Robert Wood Johnson Foundation, 1987).

Data from NHIS are not adjusted by severity of illness. Even so, NHIS found that poor children (under age 17) had fewer physician visits than non-poor children. Poor adults (between ages 17 and 64) and the poor elderly (over age 64) had a higher average number of such visits per year than the non-poor in the same age ranges; however, it has long been established that the poor have a significantly higher burden of illness than the non-poor (National Center for Health Statistics, 1988).

Ethnicity, location, education, and social circumstances contribute to difficulties in obtaining needed medical care, but the primary reason for access problems among the poor and near-poor is financial. Obviously, the inability to pay for care is a condition that also applies to the homeless poor (Robertson and Cousineau, 1986). Nine percent of low-income people reported to the Johnson surveyors instances in which they had been deterred from seeking medical care for financial reasons or had sought care and had been turned away (Freeman et al., 1987). Predictably, the greatest difficulties in obtaining medical care are experienced by low-income people without health insurance, either public or private. As shown in Figure 4-1, the proportion of those deterred from care by financial considerations is twice as great (13 percent) among the uninsured as that among the population as a whole (6 percent).

The most likely explanation for the Johnson survey's finding of reduced access to health care compared with that 5 years ago, especially for low-income Americans, is the substantial increase in the number of people without health insurance. Although the numbers are subject to interpretation and are not derived from entirely consistent data sources, the number of Americans without health insurance at any given time has increased from roughly 25 million in 1977 to perhaps as many as 37 million or 38 million today. Slightly more than half of the uninsured live in households with incomes that are less than 150 percent of the poverty level. More than half of the uninsured live in households that have at least one employed person (Sulvetta and Swartz, 1986). In addition, as Table 4-1 indicates, those people without health insurance coverage are concentrated primarily in the younger segment of the U.S. population

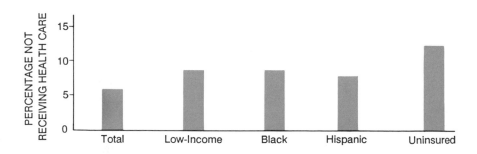

FIGURE 4-1 Percentage of Americans not receiving health care for economic reasons in 1986. SOURCE: Kovar (1987).

TABLE 4-1   Health Insurance Coverage, Fourth Quarter, 1985 (numbers in thousands)

Age and Race	Population	Percentage Covered by Insurance	No. not Covered by Insurance	Percentage not Covered by Insurance	Percent Distribution of Uncovered Population
Total	235,520	86.7	31,285	13.3	100.0
Age					
<16	55,612	84.5	8,616	15.5	27.5
16–24	34,596	78.6	7,389	21.4	23.6
25–34	41,363	83.6	6,786	16.4	21.7
35–44	32,133	89.1	3,514	10.9	11.2
45–54	22,459	90.0	2,273	10.1	7.3
55–64	22,135	88.5	2,553	11.5	8.2
Total under 65	208,298	85.1	31,131	14.9	99.5
Total 65 and over	27,222	99.4	154	0.6	0.5
Race					
White	200,083	87.6	24,840	12.4	79.4
Black	28,496	80.7	5,501	19.3	17.6
Spanish origin[a]	14,175	73.0	3,822	27.0	12.2

NOTE: Numbers do not add due to rounding.

[a]People of Spanish origin may be of either race.

SOURCE: U.S. Bureau of the Census (1985).

and among minorities, two subpopulations that are disproportionately represented among the homeless.

Here, the NHIS data tend to support the Johnson survey, at least concerning the extent of the problem of a lack of health insurance among the poor. NHIS reported that 28 percent of families with an annual income below $10,000 lacked any form of health insurance, even Medicaid. Because NHIS found that virtually all respondents in their survey who were over age 65 had some coverage (usually Medicare, frequently with some supplemental coverage), the more accurate figure for those with incomes below $10,000 per year is that for the poor population under age 65. When the elderly are removed from the calculation, the proportion of the poor without any coverage rises to 32 percent for those with incomes under $5,000 per year and to 37 percent for those with incomes between $5,000 and $9,999 per year. According to NHIS, among those under age 65, the groups most likely to lack coverage (irrespective of income) are those who are unemployed (38 percent), the poor (35 percent), those with less than 12 years of education (26 percent), those between the ages of 18 and 24 (25 percent), and blacks and others (20 percent each). As to why people lack coverage, 63 percent of the respondents to the NHIS survey who did not have coverage identified the inability to afford such insurance as their primary reason (U.S. Department of Health and Human Services, 1987).

For the proportion of uninsured people to be so great and to be increasing appears to be unprecedented in recent history. Although the number of uninsured people increased with the growth of unemployment during the recession of 1981–1982 (as was the case in earlier recessions), it has continued to increase during the period of economic growth that has largely prevailed since then. Beginning in the 1930s, economic growth in the United States has invariably been accompanied by expanded and improved health insurance coverage (along with other employment-based fringe benefits), but that pattern no longer holds. As Table 4-2 indicates, the percentage of uninsured has steadily increased since 1980 (there was a slight decrease of 0.2 percent in 1986).

Over the past several decades, health insurance has been tied primarily to employment for most nonelderly Americans or to income support programs through Medicaid for those outside the labor market. The growth in the number of uninsured people during the past decade has occurred largely among the employed, and may be attributable to changes in the labor market. Employment in manufacturing industries, which have traditionally provided the most generous insurance benefits, has fallen, and the most dramatic employment increases have occurred in service industries in which employee benefits have historically been and continue to be less generous. In addition, although the unemployment

TABLE 4-2 Nonelderly Population Without Health Insurance, 1980–1986

Year	Nonelderly Population (in millions)	No. of Nonelderly Uninsured (in millions)	Percentage Uninsured
1980	199.0	29.6	14.9
1981	200.6	NA[a]	NA
1982	202.1	30.7	15.2
1983	203.9	32.7	16.0
1984	205.6	35.0	17.0
1985	207.2	36.8	17.8
1986	209.4	36.9	17.6

[a]NA = Not available.

SOURCE: U.S. Congress, House, Committee on Ways and Means (1987).

rate has fallen in the past several years, the labor force has expanded dramatically, so that the *number* of unemployed people remains quite sizable.

Among low-income people, access to health care is often difficult, even for those who have Medicaid coverage or private insurance. Access to health care is still more difficult for people without any form of health insurance. Extending health insurance to those not presently covered is a critical issue in terms of preventing homelessness, especially as it may result from the financial consequences of illness or injury. As indicated earlier, one principal barrier to care is financial, but other barriers include an undersupply of services in many poor communities, provider hostility or resistance, cultural differences, and transportation.

This last barrier—transportation—is especially crucial for the rural poor. Transportation to and from health care facilities in rural areas may be largely unavailable, and clinics may be located many miles away. During the site visits to rural areas in Alabama, Minnesota, Mississippi, and North Dakota, members of the committee heard references to poor people in need of health care paying a friend or neighbor to transport them to a health care program, with no guarantee of a return trip home. Health care could literally be out of reach for the rural poor and the rural homeless.

Both the health care system for the indigent and the Medicaid system impose considerable noneconomic costs on their users as a result of resource scarcity, governmental suspicion of the beneficiaries of public programs, or both. Waiting times are often long at hospital clinics or income maintenance eligibility centers; physical amenities are generally few; and the hours of operation often appear to have been established to suit the convenience of the facilities' employees rather than that of its clients. These problems are encountered by many low-income people, but they have especially severe consequences for the homeless.

MEDICAID

In the United States, the major program for the provision of health insurance for low-income people now covers a smaller fraction of the poor than it did at any time in the past decade. Aggregate Medicaid enrollment has not grown, but the number of poor people has increased by roughly 40 percent (U.S. Department of Health and Human Services, 1985). To understand the importance and limitations of Medicaid as a vehicle for providing access to health care for low-income people, including the homeless, it is necessary to penetrate a thicket of Medicaid practices, beginning with two of Medicaid's fundamental precepts: eligibility and benefits.

Eligibility

Medicaid was erected on the structures of the preexisting income maintenance programs provided under the Social Security Act, specifically, Aid to Families with Dependent Children (AFDC) and Aid to the Blind, the Disabled, and the Old-Aged, all of which (except AFDC) were federalized and subsumed under Supplemental Security Income (SSI) in 1972 (Stevens and Stevens, 1974). Eligibility for either AFDC or SSI automatically confers Medicaid eligibility on the recipient, except in a few complicated instances in certain states. In addition, states may provide Medicaid for "categorically related people," those in households that would be eligible for AFDC or SSI except that their incomes exceed eligibility standards by no more than one-third. Categorically related people may also be covered, at state option, if they are "medically needy," meaning that their total income minus their medical expenses is less than a set level determined by the state. That level ranges from the maximum standard of income eligibility up to 133⅓ percent of that standard.

As with income maintenance programs, Medicaid is a federal–state program financed in part (about 54 percent) by the federal government, but administered by the states under federal rules and supervision. The latitude for state discretion is extremely wide and the result is extraordinary diversity. It is often suggested that Medicaid is best understood as 54 separate programs (the 50 states plus the District of Columbia, Puerto Rico, the Virgin Islands, and Guam), rather than a single, unitary program. Thus, individuals with incomes as high as $414 a month, before medical expenses, are eligible for Medicaid in Wisconsin, although an income in excess of $117 a month would render individuals ineligible in Tennessee. For a family of four in Alabama, $147 a month is the cutoff point for eligibility, but a family of four in California is "medically needy" at an income level of $801 per month (U.S. Department of Health and Human Services, 1985). Table 4-3 illustrates the wide diversity from state to state of the threshold of eligibility based on annual income (and percentage of the official poverty level) for the three major programs (AFDC, medically needy, and SSI) that enable a family or individual to be eligible for Medicaid. Interstate variation extends to eligibility categories as well as income levels. A particularly dramatic example is the contrast between the 27 states that provide AFDC (and thus, automatically, Medicaid) to two-parent households with children in which the principal wage earner is unemployed and the 23 states in which such households are ineligible for Medicaid (U.S. Congress, House, Committee on Ways and Means, 1987).

Perhaps of still greater concern, in terms of the problems of homeless

TABLE 4-3 Annualized Medicaid Eligibility Thresholds (AFDC, Medically Needy, SSI) as a Percentage of Poverty,[a] January 1987

State	Income ($) for AFDC Family of 3	Percentage of Poverty ($9,120[b])	Income ($) for Medically Needy Family of 3	Percentage of Poverty ($9,120[b])	Income ($) for SSI-Independent Individual[c]	Percentage of Poverty ($5,360[b])
Alabama	1,416	15.5	—	—	4,800	89.6
Alaska	8,988	78.8	—	—	7,584	113.2
Arizona	3,516	38.6	—	—	4,080	76.1
Arkansas	2,304	25.3	3,100	34.0	4,080	76.1
California	7,404	81.2	9,900	108.6	6,720	125.4
Colorado	5,052	55.4	—	—	4,776	89.1
Connecticut	6,060	66.4	7,300	80.0	5,828	108.7
Delaware	3,720	40.8	—	—	4,080	76.1
District of Columbia	4,200	46.1	5,820	63.8	4,260	79.5
Florida	3,168	34.7	4,308	47.2	4,080	76.1
Georgia	3,072	33.7	4,104	45.0	4,080	76.1
Hawaii	5,616	53.5	5,700	54.3	4,139	67.1
Idaho	3,648	40.0	—	—	4,716	88.0
Illinois	4,104	45.0	5,496	60.3	—[d]	—
Indiana	3,072	33.7	—	—	4,080	76.1
Iowa	4,572	50.1	6,096	66.8	4,080	76.1
Kansas	4,524	49.6	5,520	60.5	4,080	76.1
Kentucky	2,364	25.9	3,204	35.1	4,080	76.1
Louisiana	2,280	25.0	3,096	33.9	4,080	76.1
Maine	6,432	70.5	6,492	71.2	4,200	78.4

Maryland	4,140	45.4	4,908	53.8	4,080	76.1
Massachusetts	5,892	64.6	7,896	86.6	5,626	105.0
Michigan	5,568	61.1	6,444	70.7	4,430	82.6
Minnesota	6,384	70.0	6,384	70.0	4,500	84.0
Mississippi	4,416	48.4	—	—	4,080	76.1
Missouri	3,348	36.7	—	—	4,080	76.1
Montana	4,248	46.6	4,848	53.2	4,080	76.1
Nebraska	4,200	46.1	5,400	59.2	4,692	87.5
Nevada	3,420	37.5	—	—	4,517	84.3
New Hampshire	4,764	52.2	5,604	61.4	4,248	79.3
New Jersey	4,848	53.2	6,492	71.2	4,455	83.1
New Mexico	3,096	33.9	—	—	4,080	76.1
New York	5,964	65.4	7,400	81.1	4,943	92.2
North Carolina	3,108	34.1	4,200	46.1	4,080	76.1
North Dakota	4,452	48.8	5,220	57.2	4,080	76.1
Ohio	3,708	40.7	—	—	4,080	76.1
Oklahoma	3,720	40.8	5,004	54.8	4,848	90.4
Oregon	4,764	52.2	6,348	69.6	4,100	76.5
Pennsylvania	4,380	48.0	5,100	55.9	4,469	83.4
Rhode Island	5,664	62.1	7,600	83.3	4,754	88.7
South Carolina	4,560	50.0	3,192	35.0	4,080	76.1
South Dakota	4,392	48.2	—	—	4,260	79.5
Tennessee	4,140	45.4	2,496	27.4	4,080	76.1
Texas	2,208	24.2	3,204	35.1	4,080	76.1
Utah	8,316	91.2	6,012	65.9	4,200	78.4

(*Continued*)

TABLE 4-3 (*Continued*)

State	Income ($) for AFDC Family of 3	Percentage of Poverty ($9,120^b)	Income ($) for Medically Needy Family of 3	Percentage of Poverty ($9,120^b)	Income ($) for SSI-Independent Individual^c	Percentage of Poverty ($5,360^b)
Vermont	6,864	75.3	7,380	80.9	4,769	89.0
Virginia	3,492	38.3	4,300	47.1	4,080	76.1
Washington	5,904	64.7	6,600	73.0	4,416	82.4
West Virginia	2,988	32.8	3,480	38.2	4,080	76.1
Wisconsin	6,528	71.6	7,692	84.3	5,300	98.9
Wyoming	4,320	47.4	—	—	4,320	80.6
Average state	4,496	48.9	5,497	59.8^e	4,474	82.8

NOTE: AFDC = Aid to Families with Dependent Children; SSI = Supplemental Security Income.

[a] Based on annualized monthly maximum countable income for a family of three (AFDC, Medically Needy) and for individuals living independently (SSI).

[b] Poverty levels for Alaska and Hawaii differ from other states: Alaska—family of 3 = $11,400; family of 1 = $6,700. Hawaii—family of 3 = $10,400; family of 1 = $6,170.

[c] SSI amount for individuals living independently includes basic federal payment plus state supplemental amount where appropriate. Federal payment is $340 per month as of January 1, 1987.

[d] Illinois budgets each case individually.

[e] The percentage represents the average medically needy threshold as a percent of poverty *only for those states that have medically needy programs*. If states without medically needy programs were included in the calculation (AFDC levels would represent eligibility thresholds), the percentage would drop significantly.

SOURCE: State Medicaid Information Center, National Governors' Association, January 1987, as cited in Lee and Korenbrot (1987).

people in obtaining Medicaid, is the extraordinary confusion surrounding Medicaid eligibility for SSI recipients or those who would be Medicaid recipients were it not for differences between federal and state eligibility standards. For example, 30 states have eligibility requirements for Medicaid that are identical to the federal SSI eligibility requirements and have a single application process; 6 states have a single eligibility requirement but separate application processes; and 14 states have separate application processes and separate—and more restrictive— eligibility standards for Medicaid (U.S. Congress, House, Committee on Ways and Means, 1987).

To complicate matters still further, 29 states operate state-only programs, which cover individuals who are not eligible under federal law, entirely at state (or combined state and local) expense. Data on state-only programs are even more fragmentary and limited than data on other aspects of Medicaid, but it appears that state-only programs largely provide benefits for individuals. These programs are directed primarily to recipients of general assistance or other non-federally supported income maintenance programs and provide relatively comprehensive benefits to significant numbers of people only in New York, Illinois, and Maryland (U.S. Department of Health and Human Services, 1985).

The net result of Medicaid eligibility practices is that only slightly over half of all people with incomes below 150 percent of the poverty level are covered by Medicaid at any one time. Among the clients of the Johnson-Pew Health Care for the Homeless (HCH) projects who were seen more than once and for whom benefit status is known ($N = 10,555$), only 21 percent were participating in Medicaid (with another 5 percent participating in Medicare and 6 percent receiving some Veterans Administration benefits) (Wright and Weber, 1987). Medicaid enrollment has remained roughly constant nationwide since the late 1970s. Because the number of poor persons has increased since then, the proportion covered by Medicaid has fallen. Moreover, although the total Medicaid population has remained roughly constant, an increasing proportion of recipients consists of chronically ill elderly people in nursing homes (the largest single Medicaid expenditure) or other physically disabled, chronically impaired people (U.S. Congress, House, Committee on Ways and Means, 1987).

These aggregate figures mask enormous interstate variation. In 1982, the range of Medicaid recipients as a percentage of people below the poverty level was from 102 percent in Hawaii to 17 percent in South Dakota. In the more populous states, the percentages ranged from 72 percent in Michigan to 47 percent in Ohio to 20 percent in Texas (U.S. Department of Health and Human Services, 1985). In both 1985 and 1986, Congress took some limited steps to reverse the trend toward declining

Medicaid enrollments for pregnant women and poor children. It did this by mandating coverage of certain classes of first-time pregnant women and infants and by permitting states to decouple eligibility for Medicaid from receipt of cash assistance, thus permitting higher eligibility standards for Medicaid than for cash assistance. Data are not yet available, but only a minority of states have undertaken substantial expansions of eligibility standards, and the net increase in enrollments appears to be relatively modest (U.S. Congress, House, Committee on Ways and Means, 1987).

Benefits

A substantial body of data demonstrates that Medicaid recipients have better access to health care than do low-income people without Medicaid or other forms of health insurance, but even for those who are eligible for Medicaid, the program has limits (Rogers et al., 1982). There is considerable latitude left to the states to define covered services and to determine how those services will be paid for.

Under federal law, every state that participates in the Medicaid program must cover inpatient hospital care, hospital outpatient services, physician services, rural health clinic services, other laboratory and x-ray services, skilled nursing facilities for adults, family planning, home health care services, and nurse-midwife services, although states may impose a number of restrictions or limitations on the use of these services. Almost all participating states also provide at least some coverage for other items, such as prescription drugs, although here the patchwork of limitations and restrictions becomes more formidable (U.S. Department of Health and Human Services, 1985).

More important than coverage limitations are payment restrictions. Before 1982, states were essentially required to pay Medicare-defined costs for inpatient hospital care, and they are still required to pay cost-related rates for inpatient hospitalization and nursing homes. However, they can pay essentially whatever they choose for other services, of which the most important are physicians' services. Thus, in 1984 the Medicaid program in Connecticut paid $6.75 for a routine office visit to a specialist, New York paid $9.00, Illinois paid $10.50, California paid $12, and a relatively generous state like Wisconsin paid $15 (U.S. Department of Health and Human Services, 1985). As a result, in most of the nation, only some physicians routinely accept Medicaid patients; conversely, the availability of Medicaid coverage has done little to stem the exodus of private practitioners and other providers of health care from low-income communities. Access to care, even for those with Medicaid coverage, is particularly problematic for those needing obstetrical care, elective surgical procedures, and certain other types of specialty care, including psychiatry (Holahan, 1984). The net effect is that even when people are covered by Medicaid, they are effectively shut out of the traditional private practice fee-for-service system and must rely on the hospital system (especially the public hospital) for physician's services (Davis et al., 1981). As discussed later in this chapter, that system is already heavily involved in providing uncompensated care to the uninsured.

Medicaid and the Homeless

For homeless people, as with other low-income people, the availability of Medicaid is erratic and at least partially a function of circumstances. Single-parent families with no income other than cash assistance are generally eligible for Medicaid coverage; single individuals without children or certified disabilities generally are not. For other low-income people, it depends on such matters as the political jurisdiction in which they reside, the size and sources of their income and assets, and their skill in negotiating the bureaucratic process. As for other poor people, Medicaid coverage can be a major benefit to the homeless in removing a primary barrier to receiving health care, but it rarely solves all access problems. Many providers of health care services, especially institutions such as hospitals and free-standing health centers, certainly are more willing to serve the poor with Medicaid coverage than those without any financial resources. Yet there are shortages of health care providers (especially private physicians) in many communities occupied by high concentrations of low-income people. In addition, Medicaid generally does little to overcome such barriers as transportation cost or difficulty, cultural differences between health care providers and potential clients, or inconvenient hours or child care arrangements (Davis et al., 1981). Furthermore, when a homeless person qualifies for Medicaid as a result of receiving SSI benefits, that same homeless person who resides in a public shelter for more than 3 months in any calendar year loses the SSI eligibility and, with that, eligibility for Medicaid. The expansion of Medicaid, and especially its decoupling from other entitlement programs, could be an important step toward improving the access of low-income Americans to health care services. In many instances, however, including that of homeless people, it would probably not be a sufficient step. The homeless encounter additional barriers to the receipt of health care services that other poor people often do not.

THE INDIGENT CARE SYSTEM

Many people get care without having Medicaid, private insurance, or personal financial resources. They received medical care even before

Medicaid was enacted. Separate from the Medicaid program, but closely and increasingly tied to it, there exists in some communities a network of health care services for low-income people that is generally less than fully adequate but that provides care for some people. This system draws on a range of resources separate from Medicaid financing.

Hospitals

The most important component of this system is the several hundred public hospitals located in inner city and low-income rural areas. They are supplemented by perhaps a roughly equivalent number of voluntary (private, not-for-profit) hospitals that, in terms of location, types of patients served, and financial resources, often closely resemble public hospitals. Many of these institutions, both public and private, are teaching hospitals that have been engaged since their inception in service to the uninsured poor, both as a reflection of a general mission and as a way of ensuring an adequate supply of patients for teaching purposes.

Using 1980 data, researchers identified 1,800 community hospitals—approximately 30 percent of the nation's total—that provide 70 percent of the hospital care to the poor, including those covered by Medicaid and those for whom hospitals receive no reimbursement at all. Fewer than 1,000 hospitals provide almost half of all care to the poor. A total of 38 percent of high-volume hospitals, as compared with 28 percent of other hospitals, are public; and 13 percent are private, not-for-profit teaching hospitals. The role of hospitals in caring for poor people is indeed highly variable, but it is not inconsistent with the data to characterize 400 to 500 urban hospitals, and a similar number of rural hospitals, as the backbone of the health care system for the indigent (Feder et al., 1984).

Altogether, the nation's hospitals provide something over $6 billion a year in bad debt and charity care, primarily to low-income people, in addition to roughly $16 billion in services to Medicaid recipients (American Hospital Association, 1986). Because the numbers of Medicaid-covered and non-Medicaid-covered poor people are roughly equal, these figures might be taken to imply that the Medicaid-covered poor receive two and a half times as many hospital services per capita as the non-Medicaid-covered poor. In fact, the dynamics of the eligibility criteria for the medically needy are such that people who need more expensive services are more likely to become eligible for Medicaid. However, the willingness of many hospitals to serve uncovered individuals does not provide the equivalent access to care as that which would exist under Medicaid.

Much too little is known about the characteristics of uncompensated care provided by hospitals, or the characteristics of patients who receive such care. However, several generalizations are possible. In many big cities, a substantial proportion of unreimbursed services is provided to outpatients. Hospital outpatient departments and emergency rooms provide routine medical care for thousands of poor people. Reliance on such services as principal providers of primary and specialized care has long been justly criticized in terms of its impersonality, lack of continuity, and expense. Efforts have been made in many communities to divert outpatient services from traditional clinics and emergency rooms to group practice arrangements, off-site clinics, or prepaid health plans. However, the entrenched system of outpatient and emergency room care is resilient.

Uncompensated inpatient services tend to be highly concentrated in a few diagnoses and types of cases, especially maternity and trauma services (Sloan and Valvona, 1986). Relatively little uncompensated care takes the form of elective surgery. For example, uninsured people who are seriously injured in automobile accidents or who have gone into labor are more likely to get inpatient hospital care than those with cataracts or chronic hernias.

There is much discussion of uncompensated hospital services being financed by shifting the costs to paying patients. In fact, the primary subsidies supporting the provision of hospital care to nonpaying patients have long come from local and state governments, from philanthropy, and from medical education. Most hospitals that provide high volumes of care to nonpaying patients have relatively small proportions of patients who pay more than their own way on whom to shift costs (Hadley and Feder, 1985). The most generous and systematic subsidization of uncompensated care takes place in six states—Connecticut, Maine, Maryland, Massachusetts, New Jersey, and New York—where such subsidies are both generated and allocated through a hospital rate-regulation mechanism. In several other states, including Florida, Nevada, and South Carolina, subventions of hospital revenues are also applied to generate revenue for subsidization of hospital-provided uncompensated care. Despite this, the National Association of Public Hospitals (NAPH) reports that 7 of the 90 major public hospitals have closed their doors in the last decade and that 50 percent of all public hospitals are running at a deficit. The NAPH attributes this to three factors: declining public payments (e.g., state and local subsidies have declined 15 percent and Medicare revenues have declined 17 percent); more indigent patients (there was a 9 percent increase in the use of outpatient departments and emergency rooms by uninsured patients between 1983 and 1985; slightly more than half of all such visits were by uninsured or self-pay patients, a quarter of which were written off as bad debt); and the rising cost of treating AIDS (acquired immune deficiency syndrome) (National Association of Public Hospitals, 1987). With regard to the last point, the National

Commission to Prevent Infant Mortality cites the increase in the number of "boarder babies"—many of whom are infants with AIDS for whom there are no homes (their own or foster homes), who, as a consequence, spend weeks or months in hospitals—as a factor in increased costs to such facilities (Medicine and Health, 1987).

Whatever the sources or magnitude of financing for uncompensated care, they have not grown over the last decade nearly as fast as the number of uninsured people has. It appears that the provision of uncompensated care by hospitals is more sensitive to the supply of the subsidy than to the demand for services. As a result, the amount of uncompensated care provided by hospitals, although it has increased substantially in the past several years, has not increased as fast as the number of uninsured people (Feder et al., 1984). Therefore, uninsured homeless individuals are, in a sense, competing with the growing numbers of other uninsured domiciled people for the relatively scarce resource of subsidized hospital services, especially because the homeless population is concentrated in those areas where the demands on hospitals are greatest.

Clinics

The other principal pillar of the indigent care system has been the free-standing clinics supported by public or philanthropic funds. These sprang up in many cities contemporaneously with the founding of modern hospitals around the turn of the century and retained a special focus on service to the poor.

The expansion of free-standing clinic services for low-income communities was encouraged by the war on poverty in the 1960s, which supported the development of about 125 neighborhood health centers serving approximately 1.5 million people. In 1976 federal support for such centers was merged with various other forms of categorical support for clinic activities under Section 330 of the Public Health Service Act (Davis and Schoen, 1978). Under the Omnibus Budget Reconciliation Act of 1981 (P.L. 97-35), federal financial support both for community-based health centers and specialized maternal and child health care centers was substantially reduced. A number of localities closed or consolidated facilities. Many health centers, public and private, were forced to reduce their budgets and services. Nonetheless, several hundred such centers survive, in both urban and rural areas, supported by federal and local—and in some instances, state—appropriations, as well as Medicaid and Medicare revenues. The performances of such centers are as diverse and variable as all their other characteristics, but most evaluations have been relatively positive. In most instances they do not appear to have supplanted hospital emergency rooms or clinics as providers of care to the poor, but rather to have reached previously unserved populations, and they remain important to the care of indigents in many communities. Few such centers reached out to the homeless before the initiation of the Robert Wood Johnson Foundation-Pew Memorial Trust Health Care for the Homeless program. However, many now constitute important components of health care services for homeless individuals.

The National Health Service Corps

Over the past decade, many of the facilities and programs that conduct health care for the medically indigent have relied on the National Health Service Corps (NHSC) for the recruitment of professional personnel. The NHSC was established in 1974 both as a response to the problems of inadequate physician supply in underserved areas and a perceived need to subsidize professional education for students who might be attracted to serve in those areas. It is now being phased out in the face of budgetary pressures and a perceived physician surplus. The NHSC has placed physicians, nurse practitioners, dentists, and other health care personnel in neighborhood health centers, free-standing clinics, outpatient departments, and other providers of service to medically underserved communities. In several of the sites visited by the committee where health care services were being provided to homeless people, NHSC practitioners played a central role. The overall performance and cost-effectiveness of the NHSC are matters of some dispute, but the committee is pleased to note that the Stewart B. McKinney Homeless Assistance Act of 1987 (P.L. 100-77) contains specific provisions authorizing NHSC placements in sites providing health care to homeless people.

Categorical Programs

Contributing further to the organizational complexities of providing care to low-income persons are hundreds of specialty outpatient programs that offer such services as family planning, alcohol and drug treatment, mental health care, disease-specific services, or services to specific populations, such as migrant workers or native Americans. While some of these programs were not designed specifically to serve the poor, they do, in effect, provide service to low-income people who are members of those groups to whom the programs are targeted. Many of these programs rely heavily on federal funding. In many instances this source of funding has been cut back in the last decade, with some substitution of state or local funding. The availability of any such services and their relevance to the needs of homeless people vary considerably from community to community, and an accurate generalization is impossible. Such service programs are, however, an important part of the indigent care system in some areas and should not be overlooked in any overview of that system.

ADDITIONAL BARRIERS TO ACCESS FOR HOMELESS PEOPLE

In their evaluation of the benefit status of homeless people seen in 16 of the Robert Wood Johnson Foundation-Pew Memorial Trust Health Care for the Homeless (HCH) projects, Wright and Weber (1987) noted that a determination of benefit status could not be made for 24 percent of the people seen by workers in these projects. Of the 76 percent for whom benefit status was known, about half were receiving some form of financial benefit and about half were not. They concluded that almost all clients of the HCH projects who were eligible for any benefits from public entitlement programs were already enrolled in them and that those who were not enrolled were not simply because they were not eligible. After examining several possible factors that conceivably could affect whether a homeless person receives any existing form of financial assistance (including Medicaid), they concluded that by far the most significant factor was the leniency of eligibility requirements for each program as determined by each state:

The "entitlement problem" for the homeless is not that they do not participate in programs for which they are eligible, but that in many states they are not eligible for programs of assistance regardless of their rather obvious needs. (Wright and Weber, 1987)

Wright and Weber noted that among the 16 projects included in their study, the proportion of homeless clients receiving any benefits ranged from 22 to 82 percent; the basis for this variation was primarily the eligibility standards of the respective states. However, they also noted that "the benefit levels typical of most social welfare programs are so low as to make only a marginal contribution" to the ultimate goal of "getting the client off the streets or out of the shelters and into some reasonably stable housing and social situation."

Ineligibility is only one barrier to access for the homeless; there are others. The extreme case of such barriers to the homeless has been the requirement that individuals have a permanent address for Medicaid eligibility or for receipt of services from certain providers with defined areas of geographic responsibility. Even with the recent passage of federal legislation prohibiting the requirement of a fixed address as a basis for eligibility for entitlement programs, homeless people are still in no position to receive mail notices of clinic appointments, laboratory or x-ray results, or required reappearances for recertification of Medicaid eligibility or appeals of disability determinations. Absence of an address is not the only documentation problem encountered by homeless people. In the shelters and on the streets, where homeless people spend much of their time, personal identification papers are a valuable commodity sought by thieves and entrepreneurs. The exigencies of a homeless existence rarely afford a means of protecting personal documents from theft, loss, or damage from the elements.

Particular problems that bureaucratic obstacles can create for homeless people were frequently reported to the committee during its site visits. One important example is the scheduling of clinic appointments and ancillary services at times that conflict with the availablity of the only daytime meals homeless people can get or with the time they must begin lining up for shelters to ensure that they have a place to sleep that night. The problems of access put a premium on the ability of homeless people to cope with and manage complicated bureaucratic systems and routines. Those abilities are often limited among homeless people in general and not only among those whose capacity is impaired by mental disorders or substance abuse. For example, the lack of a watch can make the keeping of appointments quite difficult. The use of public transportation, a frequent source of frustration even for the average urban commuter, presents a greater impediment to a person who has money for only one fare and cannot afford to make mistakes in matters of transfers or routes. Moreover, providers experienced in working with homeless people report that they avoid institutions and bureaucratic procedures, often because of prior negative experiences (Brickner et al., 1985). In addition, in many instances service providers are not interested in efforts to reduce these barriers. Homeless people can appear as extremely unattractive potential clients that institutions or professionals may try to avoid. At the most basic level, homeless people often are physically unattractive, unwashed, and lack clean clothes. They may not be compliant, in part because of the exigencies of a homeless existence. Providers often feel that they will not or cannot follow through with therapeutic or self-care regimens (Brickner et al., 1985).

Many homeless people, with or without identifiable mental illness, are passively resistant to service provision, including health services (Vicic and Doherty, 1987). Successfully engaging such persons for purposes of diagnosis and treatment involves extra efforts on the part of health care providers. Many providers may not be sufficiently motivated or knowl-edgeable to undertake such efforts. The health care system in general, and providers of service to poor people in particular, are most responsive to those patients who are most motivated, demanding, or both. Providers of services tend to react negatively to those who appear to be uncooperative or uncompliant.

MENTAL HEALTH CARE

Approximately one-third of all homeless people show symptoms of mental illness. The barriers to access discussed above generally apply also to this group of homeless people. In most respects, especially with regard to the reluctance of health care institutions and providers to treat the homeless, the barriers are even greater.

There are, however, two major exceptions to this observation. The mentally ill among the homeless are theoretically more likely than those without such a disability to be eligible for SSI benefits (and, therefore, Medicaid). The SSI program specifically provides for benefits to the mentally disabled. This greater access to SSI eligibility is, however, somewhat illusory because the standards by which disability is determined are open to a wide range of interpretations. The extent to which such interpretations can determine eligibility was clearly seen during 1981–1984 when, in response to what was intended to be simply a clarification of such standards, thousands of mentally disabled people were dropped from the SSI rolls. Later restoration of most of them did not completely allay misgivings about the operation.

The potential of the mentally ill for SSI eligibility may be helpful, but the health care benefits received to support treatment for mental illness are generally inadequate, if not inappropriate. In those states in which Medicaid programs fund mental health care (not all do), it is usually only for inpatient care, and then it is only for a very limited period of time (usually 30 days). The prospective patient, therefore, is in a situation of being declared eligible for benefits based on a disability for which treatment is either poorly funded or not funded at all. The concept that such treatment might ultimately enable the individual to move on to productive employment appears to have been sacrificed to cost-containment measures.

Government, especially at the state level, has long accepted a primary responsibility for the provision of mental health services. The creation of large state-operated mental health facilities goes back to the middle 1800s, and many states mandate such a responsibility in their state constitutions. A role for the federal government is more recent, having largely begun with the report of the Joint Commission on Mental Illness and Health, *Action for Mental Health,* in 1961 and the various pieces of legislation that sought to implement the most significant recommendations of that commission. The general intent of that legislation was to transfer mental health care from the large state-operated hospitals to small community-based mental health centers. This, as much as the discovery and widespread use of psychotropic drugs, was a key element in what is now called deinstitutionalization.

At the time of passage of the Mental Retardation Facilities and Community Mental Health Centers Construction Act of 1963 (P.L. 88-184), it was anticipated that 2,500 community mental health centers would be constructed throughout the United States. At best, only about 700 of these centers ever opened (President's Commission on Mental Health, 1978). Unlike the general health care system, which has a seemingly adequate supply of hospitals, the mental health care system severely lacks the most basic units for treatment—posing the ultimate barrier to access.

Despite substantial increases in state spending on mental health, little has been done to increase the supply of community-based mental health care centers. Of the approximately $6 billion spent annually on state-operated mental health care, more than $4 billion, or approximately 70 percent, is spent on state institutions (Rubenstein, 1986). Although to some extent this allocation of expenditures is the result of the effort to upgrade the quality of care in state institutions that accompanied the effort to transfer care to community-based facilities, the net effect on the mentally ill person in the community remains the same: there is no place to go. In the competition for such a scarce resource as community-based treatment, the homeless person is in a particularly uncompetitive position.

There have been some recent developments toward increasing access to mental health care services for the homeless. One of the most notable programs is the Community Support Program (CSP), which is directed by the National Institute of Mental Health. CSP was developed to provide time-limited demonstration grants in support of efforts to find new approaches for providing services to the homeless mentally ill. The Stewart B. McKinney Homeless Assistance Act of 1987 (P.L. 100-77) authorized an additional $10 million for this program for fiscal year 1987 as well as $30 million for a new block grant program for services to homeless people who are chronically mentally ill.

The mentally ill among the homeless are quite noticeable, and this has raised anew old issues regarding a civil commitment to treatment facilities. The current basis of commitment in most states can be described as a clear and present danger to him- or herself or others. Even in those states that have a broader basis for commitment (e.g., an inability to perform life-sustaining activities), such factors as budget constraints, fear of legal reaction, or a desire to provide treatment in the least restrictive environment have left the clear and present danger criterion as the basis for commitment. As a consequence, a new approach, outpatient commitment, has been proposed (American Psychiatric Association, 1987). Outpatient commitment refers to the procedure by which a court orders treatment in the community for a person who does not meet the standard for civil commitment to an institution (Kanter, 1987). Such an approach is based on an assumption that there are programs in existence that are not only prepared to treat people so committed but that have the facilities and space to do so. That is not the case in most jurisdictions. Especially troublesome are reports of attempts to commit mentally ill people to outpatient services and then require that they pay for those services (Stefan, 1986). The penalties that would be imposed on someone who is committed by the courts to outpatient services and who then refused to pay for such services have not yet been identified.

VETERANS

As many as 40 percent of the homeless adult men in some communities are veterans, and many of those are Vietnam-era veterans. Some may be eligible for services from the largest public health care system in the United States: the Veterans Administration (VA).

The VA health care system includes 172 hospitals, 229 outpatient clinics, 117 nursing homes, 16 domiciliary facilities, and a range of contracted services, directly employing more than 200,000 people at an annual expense of almost $10 billion. In fiscal year 1986, this system provided almost 1.5 million inpatient stays and more than 20 million outpatient visits. It has particularly extensive services for alcoholism and drug dependence, operating 103 specialized alcoholism programs and 51 specialty drug dependence programs (Veterans Administration, 1987).

Veterans with an unblemished discharge status are automatically eligible for free VA services for the treatment of service-connected illnesses or disabilities; free or subsidized services are also available to low-income and elderly veterans. Although they are more stringent than they have been in the past, the income eligibility criteria for VA medical services remain substantially more generous than those of other publicly supported benefits.

Yet, it is widely believed that relatively few homeless people take advantage of the VA health care services to which they are at least theoretically entitled. In part as a response to this perception, the VA has undertaken a number of initiatives to expand services to homeless veterans. Five million dollars has been appropriated for 43 demonstration projects for the community-based treatment of the chronically mentally ill, with particular emphasis on outreach to homeless veterans. Additional funds were appropriated in mid-1987 for the development of new and expanded domiciliary services for homeless veterans, and a number of VA facilities and programs have begun to undertake more aggressive outreach programs to homeless veterans, as mandated by the Omnibus Budget Reconciliation Act of 1986 (P.L. 99-509).

The interim report of that effort, released in October 1987 and covering the first 4 months of the Homeless Chronically Mentally Ill (HCMI) outreach project, partially confirmed the belief that homeless veterans do not—for various reasons—avail themselves of VA medical services (Rosenheck et al., 1987). Although 97 percent of the 6,342 individuals contacted during the first 4 months appeared to be eligible veterans (i.e., veterans who had been honorably discharged), of those for whom intake assessments were completed ($N = 4,010$), only 18 percent were receiving any financial support from the VA. With regard to access to VA health and mental health care, a sample of 727 veterans contacted through the HCMI program showed that 75 percent of the sample had three or fewer contacts with VA mental health outpatient services during the 6 months immediately prior to contact with the outreach program; 42 percent had no contact with any medical or psychiatric outpatient providers, but 38 percent did have at least one admission to some form of inpatient care.

VA health care facilities are often located at some distance from where homeless people congregate. This presents a serious issue of access, especially if there is no specific outreach program to homeless veterans. This situation is further exacerbated by the VA's system of priority eligibility; who actually receives care is based on the level of disability, whether it is service connected, and the capacity of the specific VA facility in question (U.S. Department of Health and Human Services, 1987). The recent initiatives of the VA are particularly encouraging, but the gap between current and potential services to homeless veterans remains considerable. In addition, the extent of the disability by which one qualifies for full benefits has been raised, making it more difficult for some veterans to qualify. Unless such veterans live in a state where their disability qualifies them for Medicaid, they may be without health care benefits. One especially troublesome issue was reported to the committee during its site visits: Veterans whose disabilities are such that they receive no or only partial VA benefits may be denied non-VA benefits (Medicaid, SSI, or general assistance), on the erroneous assumption, by those responsible for determining eligibility for non-VA programs, that the financial relief for such individuals should come from the VA. The VA HCMI project found that more than half (54.8 percent) of the veterans seen in the sample of intake assessments were receiving no benefits from any source.

One final—and substantial—barrier to access to care for veterans comes in the nature of their discharge from military service. If their military discharge was anything other than honorable (i.e., less than honorable or dishonorable), they are effectively barred from receiving VA benefits.

The VA has a system by which the nature of a discharge can be reviewed and possibly upgraded, but it is cumbersome and requires extensive documentation. It is also not well publicized among veterans, especially disaffiliated homeless veterans. Each of these are specific and serious obstacles to the receipt of health care services by homeless veterans. Outreach and educational programs, such as those that are now being initiated by the VA, as well as counseling programs, which have been conducted for many years by such organizations as Vietnam Veterans of America and Swords to Plowshares, could be highly effective in resolving veterans' access to health care. Ultimately, the success of such efforts depends on the criteria—and the interpretation of those criteria—by which requisites for upgrading of discharge status will be evaluated.

SUMMARY

Homeless people, who are predominantly low-income, uninsured residents of mostly low-income communities, share with other low-income residents of such communities a range of difficulties in getting health care when they need it. The most significant barriers to access are financial. At the same time, the homeless encounter a range of additional barriers to health care.

In order to develop service programs to meet the health care needs of homeless people, it is necessary to address both the general issues of access to care and the special problems encountered by homeless people in obtaining access. Financing mechanisms are obviously the first precondition, whether they are through improving eligibility for Medicaid or other benefit programs or through procurement of direct subsidies. Financing, however, while a necessary condition, is not sufficient. Problems of scheduling, transportation, and negotiating systems must also be solved. The practices and attitudes of providers, along with the special problems posed by the passivity, isolation, and resistance of homeless people, many of whom have had negative experiences with health care institutions, must also be taken into consideration. How some of these problems have been met in a number of specific programs is the primary content of the next chapter.

REFERENCES

Aday, L. A., G. V. Fleming, and R. Andersen. 1984. Access to Medical Care in the U.S.: Who Has It, Who Doesn't. Chicago: Pluribus Press.

American Hospital Association. 1986. Hospital Statistics: 1985. Chicago: American Hospital Association.

American Psychiatric Association. 1987. Involuntary Commitment to Outpatient Treatment: Report of the Task Force on Involuntary Outpatient Commitment. Task force report no. 26. Washington, D.C.: American Psychiatric Association.

Brickner, P. W., L. K. Scharer, B. Conanan, A. Elvy, and M. Savarese, eds. 1985. Health Care of Homeless People. New York: Springer-Verlag.

Davis, K., and C. Schoen. 1978. Health and the War on Poverty: A Ten-Year Appraisal. Washington, D.C.: Brookings Institution.

Davis, K., M. Gold, and D. Makuc. 1981. Access to health care for the poor: Does the gap remain? Annual Review of Public Health 2:159–182.

Feder, J., J. Hadley, and R. Mullner. 1984. Poor people and poor hospitals: Implications for public policy. Journal of Health Politics, Policy and Law 9(2):237–250.

Freeman, H. E., R. J. Blendon, L. H. Aiken, S. Sudman, C. F. Mullinix, and C. R. Corey. 1987. Americans report on their access to care. Health Affairs 6(1):6–18.

Hadley, J., and J. Feder. 1985. Hospital cost shifting and care for the uninsured. Health Affairs 4(3):67–80.

Holahan, J. 1984. Paying for physician services in state Medicaid programs. Health Care Financing Administration Review 5(3):99–110.

Joint Commission on Mental Illness and Health. 1961. Action for Mental Health: Final Report. New York: Basic Books.

Kanter, A. S. 1987. Legal barriers to access: The unmet health care needs of homeless people. Mental Health Law Project, Washington, D.C. Paper prepared for the Institute of Medicine, Washington, D.C.

Kovar, M. G. 1987. Letter to the publisher: Questioning the reported decline in use of ambulatory care. Health Affairs 6(Winter):156–157.

Lee, P., and C. Korenbrot. 1987. The Prevention of Low-Weight Births: A Policy Research Analysis. San Francisco: Institute for Health Policy Studies, University of California, San Francisco.

Medicine and Health. 1987. Panel seeks help for AIDS babies. Medicine and Health 41(44):2.

National Association of Public Hospitals. 1987. America's Health Safety Net. Washington, D.C.: National Association of Public Hospitals.

National Center for Health Statistics. 1988. Health Interview Survey. National Center for Health Statistics, Washington, D.C. (Unpublished.)

New York Times. December 1, 1987. Poll finds Reagan support down but Democrats still lacking fire. A1.

President's Commission on Mental Health. 1978. P. 319 in Task Panel Reports Submitted to the President's Commission on Mental Health, Volume II, Appendix. Washington, D.C.: U.S. Government Printing Office.

President's Commission for the Study of Ethical Problems in Medicine and Biomedical and Behavioral Research. 1983. Securing Access to Health Care: The Ethical Implications of Differences in the Availability of Health Services, Volume 1: Report. Washington, D.C.: U.S. Government Printing Office.

Robert Wood Johnson Foundation. 1987. Special Report on Access to Medical Care, no. 2. Princeton, N.J.: Robert Wood Johnson Foundation.

Robertson, M. J., and M. R. Cousineau. 1986. Health status and access to health services among the urban homeless. American Journal of Public Health 76(5):561–563.

Rogers, D. E., R. J. Blendon, and T. W. Moloney. 1982. Who needs Medicaid? New England Journal of Medicine 307(1):13–18.

Rosenheck, R., P. Gallup, C. Leda, P. Leaf, R. Milstein, I. Voynick, P. Errera, L. Lehman, G. Koerber, and R. Murphy. 1987. Progress Report on the Veterans Administration Program for Homeless Chronically Mentally Ill Veterans. Washington, D.C.: Veterans Administration.

Rubenstein, L. 1986. Access to treatment and rehabilitation for severely mentally ill poor people. Clearinghouse Review 20(4):382–393.

Sloan, F. A., and J. Valvona. 1986. Uncovering the high costs of teaching hospitals. Health Affairs 5(3):68–85.

Stefan, S. 1986. Outpatient Commitment Evaluation of Criteria and Programs. (Unpublished; see also Kanter, A. S. 1987.)

Stevens, R., and R. Stevens. 1974. Welfare Medicine in America: A Case Study of Medicaid. New York: The Free Press.

Sulvetta, M., and K. Swartz. 1986. The Uninsured and Uncompensated Care: A Chartbook. Washington, D.C.: National Health Policy Forum, George Washington University.

U.S. Bureau of the Census. 1985. Disability, Functional Limitation, and Health Insurance Coverage: 1984/85. Series P-70, No. 8, Table 10. Current Population Reports. Washington, D.C.: U.S. Government Printing Office. (Cited in U.S. Congress, House, Committee on Ways and Means, 1987, p. 218.)

U.S. Congress, House, Committee on Ways and Means. 1987. Background material and data on programs within the jurisdiction of the Committee on Ways and Means. 100th Cong., 1st sess., March 6, 1987.

U.S. Congressional Budget Office. 1986. Tabulations of current population surveys, March 1980–March 1986. Washington, D.C.: U.S. Government Printing Office. (Cited in U.S. Congress, House, Committee on Ways and Means, 1987, p. 219.)

U.S. Department of Health and Human Services. 1985. Health Care Financing Program Statistics: Analysis of State Medicaid Program Characteristics, 1984. Baltimore: Office of the Actuary, Health Care Financing Administration.

U.S. Department of Health and Human Services. 1987. Health Care Coverage by Age, Sex, Race and Family Income: United States, 1986. Vital and Health Statistics, No. 139, September 18, 1987. Washington, D.C.: National Center for Health Statistics.

Veterans Administration. 1987. Annual Report: 1986. Washington, D.C.: U.S. Government Printing Office

Vicic, W. J., and P. Doherty, 1987. Homelessness: A Medical Viewpoint. Paper prepared for the Institute of Medicine, Washington, D.C.

Wright, J. D., and E. Weber. 1987. Homelessness and Health. New York: McGraw-Hill.

5

Health Care Services for Homeless People

INTRODUCTION

To the extent that homeless people have been able to obtain needed health care services, they have relied on emergency rooms, clinics, hospitals, and other facilities that serve the poor. Indigent people (with or without a home) experience many obstacles in obtaining health care. For homeless people there are additional barriers. Recognition of the special health care needs of homeless people has encouraged the development of special services for them. In observing and describing these health care and health care-related services, one must be mindful of the heterogeneous nature of the homeless population, as well as the structure of the communities in which such services have developed. Regardless of differences among homeless people or regional variations in services, however, homeless people are more susceptible to certain diseases, have greater difficulty getting health care, and are harder to treat than other people, all because they lack a home. Similarly, attempts to provide health and mental health care services, regardless of variations in such areas as history, funding levels, and nature of support, also have certain common elements. They arose in response to a crisis rather than developing as part of a well thought out plan. They generally brought services *to* homeless people rather than waiting for them to come in; increasingly, they rely on public funding because the problem has grown beyond a level that the private sector can support.

The purpose of this chapter is to describe programs that seek to bring general health and mental health care services to homeless people. The information presented in this chapter is largely based on the 11 site visits

103

made by members of the study committee and its staff. Although the sites are not representative of the entire universe of programs for the homeless, they were selected to include the broadest range of programs possible and to be geographically dispersed throughout the country.

In studying health care and related services for homeless people, the committee sought to examine a broad range of services developed over a period of time, rather than to focus only on specialized services or services that have been developed recently. However, what the committee observed were discrete services and programs. At no time did the committee encounter anything that could be appropriately called a "system" of services.

Before describing how these various programs bring general health care and mental health care to the homeless, we must address two major issues: (1) what makes serving the homeless, in contrast to the indigent in general, more difficult?; and (2) based upon the literature and the site visits, what elements enhance a program's ability to provide such services to this population? In Chapter 3, we discussed those aspects of treatment that are especially difficult to implement when the patient is homeless. However, one must also look at the people who are homeless. William Breakey (in press) has identified characteristics of homeless people that affect the provision of treatment and the planning of health care services:

Daily Activities—Some homeless people live under circumstances that pose particular problems for developing a treatment plan. For many, it may be difficult to keep a supply of medication while living on the street. For an alcoholic trying to stay sober, a homeless existence may present too many opportunities for drinking. Some former patients complain that neuroleptic medications, prescribed for a schizophrenic illness, may make them too drowsy and interfere with their alertness against the dangers on the streets.

Multiplicity of Needs—In addition to physical and mental health problems and difficulties with such things as housing and income maintenance, homeless people often also suffer from drug or alcohol abuse. Any health care program for homeless adults should expect that 25 to 40 percent of patients will suffer from serious alcohol or drug abuse problems (Fischer and Breakey, 1986).

Disaffiliation—Although many homeless people establish individual support networks outside a family structure, some homeless people typically lack those networks that enable most people to sustain themselves in society. Such isolation often causes (and sometimes is caused by) a limited capacity to establish supportive relationships with other people. Difficulties in establishing and maintaining relationships can militate against the development of cooperation with health care providers and may be an important factor in explaining what is often inaccurately described as a "lack of motivation."

Distrust—In addition to their distrust of authority, many homeless people are disenchanted with health and mental health care providers. Some have had bad experiences with medications, hospitals, doctors, and other human service professionals and are leery of further involvement.

Except for anecdotal information and obvious indicators of utilization, it is not possible to assess the effectiveness of health care delivery systems for homeless people. There are no adequate data from which such assessments can be made. However, in its review of various programs for health and mental health care services for homeless people, the committee found that four common elements enhanced a program's ability to provide services to this population:

Communication—Those people and agencies involved in the effort to address the health care problems of homeless people interact regularly and frequently.

Coordination—Even if only in a most rudimentary form, there is some way in which clients can be linked with a wide range of existing services (i.e., health and mental health care, housing, social services, entitlements, etc.) by providers, rather than being forced to seek services without assistance.

Targeted Approach—Programs are aggressive in seeking the homeless, rather than passive in waiting for them to appear. This may be reflected by locating a program in a skid row area. Other programs provide outreach and seek out homeless individuals on the streets.

Internal and External Resources—These constitute the range of resources that a program requires to carry out its function adequately, no matter how limited that function might be. Internal resources include reasonable funding and paid employees, in addition to the utilization of volunteers and donated goods and facilities. External resources include both the network of essential services described above and the ability to access that network.

The Health Care for the Homeless projects, funded jointly by the Robert Wood Johnson Foundation and the Pew Memorial Trust, are considered by many to have been the single most effective network of health care services developed for homeless people in the 1980s. They are also generally viewed as providing a major impetus for Title VI (health care) of the recently passed Stewart B. McKinney Homeless Assistance Act of 1987 (P.L. 100-77). The first nationwide program to address the health care problems of the homeless, the projects' creation serves as a benchmark. Therefore, this chapter is arranged from the perspective of that unique role. The following sections of this chapter describe: (1) programs in existence prior to the Johnson-Pew projects;* (2) the Johnson-Pew program itself; and (3) other programs that came into existence at

---

* The term Johnson-Pew is not generally used to describe these projects. It is used in this report because the more commonly used name of the project, Health Care for the Homeless projects, could just as easily describe many programs that are not funded by this particular grant.

roughly the same time (1984–1987) as the Johnson-Pew projects. The description of the third group is further subdivided, based upon the targeted populations. The final section of this chapter discusses various programmatic, administrative, and clinical issues identified throughout the course of the committee's observation of these service delivery models.

PRE-JOHNSON-PEW MODELS

Several program models were developed to provide health care services to homeless people before the mid-1980s. The conclusion that they are effective models of service delivery can be drawn from their reported experiences and the fact that the major features of such models appear repeatedly in later programs (especially the 19 Johnson-Pew projects).

Shelter-Based Clinics

Shelter-based clinics provide the types of services most frequently found throughout the country. Recognizing a need to bring services to where homeless people can be found, those involved with shelters or health care have developed on-site clinics at shelter locations.

Rescue Missions

The committee visited volunteer clinics located at rescue missions in Kansas City, Los Angeles, Nashville, and San Diego. These rescue missions are coordinated on the national level by the International Union of Gospel Missions, but there is an even greater strength of coordination locally. Having served the homeless for extended periods, they are known to the community and have substantial access to existing networks of, for example, health care services, housing, and social services. The clinics tend to be staffed by volunteer doctors and nurses and rely heavily on private donations, both of cash and pharmaceutical and medical supplies (although some have begun to accept limited financial support from local governments). However, because of the religious aspects of the organizations that operate these clinics, not every homeless person is willing to go to them.

Nonsectarian Programs

Nonsectarian programs, such as the clinic at the Pine Street Inn in Boston, operate similarly to the religious rescue missions. They have developed strong sources of financial support, frequently from among local businesses, charitable organizations, and foundations. In the absence of any national coordinating or controlling body, they tend to reflect the characteristics and needs of the city in which they are located.

Both the rescue missions and the nonsectarian programs face certain common problems: limited hours (many shelters are closed during the day), dependence on volunteers, limited access to some of the less common medications, limited specialty and ancillary services (e.g., podiatry and dental care), lack of an ability to perform systematic screening, and difficulty in obtaining both liability insurance and medical malpractice insurance (especially critical when volunteers are retired physicians who do not have their own malpractice insurance). Both the rescue missions and the nonsectarian programs are, however, major sources of private, not-for-profit, and non-tax-supported health care for homeless people.

The Public–Private Programs

Public–private programs share some of the attributes of all volunteer clinics, but they have often resolved some of the problems cited above. One of the oldest examples is the St. Vincent's Hospital and Medical Center Single Room Occupancy (SRO) and Shelter Program in New York City.* The initial program developed from an intern's concerns over the large number of people who arrived by ambulance from one SRO hotel. Outreach programs were designed to provide health and social services on-site at SRO hotels and municipal shelters. With some variance according to the site at which services are provided, an interdisciplinary team of a physician, a nurse, and a social worker established on-site medical clinics. In recent years, partial funding for the program has been received from the New York City Human Resources Administration, that city's department of social services. In addition to the benefits of on-site programming, the clinics and the Department of Community Services at the hospital closely coordinate their efforts. Homeless people referred to the hospital for specialized services are often treated by the same individuals whom they saw at the on-site clinic, improving the continuity of care and increasing cooperation with the care-giver.

Health Care Services in Day Programs

Day programs, which are similar to the shelter-based clinics identified above, provide services where homeless people can be found, but they differ from shelter-based clinics in that the sites are independent of

---

* For a more detailed description of the St. Vincent's program, see Brickner et al. (1985).

residential programs. One good example is St. Francis House in Boston, which has been described by its staff as "a shopping mall of services to the homeless." Various mental health and vocational guidance services are provided to homeless people in a single building located in what was once known as the "combat zone"* of Boston. Included in these services is a health clinic for homeless people that is staffed by volunteers and paid employees.

A similar program, also in Boston, is the Cardinal Medeiros Day Center operated by the Kit Clarke Senior House. Located in a church in downtown Boston, this is a day program exclusively for elderly homeless people. Among its services is a food van that stops where the elderly homeless are known to congregate. A registered nurse who is part of the van team performs basic health assessments and referrals for anyone willing to accept this service. A second nurse, stationed at the Medeiros Center, provides more extensive services. The two nurses alternate between the van and the center, so they are familiar with both programs and are readily identified by the homeless people themselves. While the nurse reported to the site visit team that there is little opportunity to perform other than the most basic visual assessment of a homeless person's health status from the van, she indicated that the true value of the program came from gaining the confidence of homeless people and then referring them to the Medeiros Center at a time when she could perform a more detailed assessment. The fact that they knew her enabled them to overcome any fear that might have prevented them from seeking health care.

A third program of this type is So Others Might Eat, known as SOME, a day program in Washington, D.C., whose primary purpose is to provide breakfast and lunch to homeless people. Since 1982, SOME has been the site for a medical clinic operated by the Columbia Road Physician Group, a group practice composed of four physicians committed to serving homeless and indigent people and providing on-site social services and substance abuse counseling. It has also been the site for a dental clinic operated by the Georgetown University Dental School.†

Free-Standing Clinics

In 1979 a somewhat different model for the delivery of health care for homeless people was started in Washington, D.C.—the Zacchaeus Clinic.

---

* The term *combat zone* came into common usage in the 1960s to describe a section of downtown Boston known as the site of strip shows, adult bookstores, and so forth. Because of its reputation as being the more "open" part of that city, it became attractive to street people. It is now undergoing commercial redevelopment.

† Both the St. Francis House and SOME, as well as the Pine Street Inn discussed earlier, have expanded in the past 2 years as the result of additional staff provided by the Johnson-Pew projects in Boston and Washington.

The clinic was funded entirely by donations from individuals, churches, community groups, and small grantors. It used a combination of paid staff and volunteers. It was established as a free-standing clinic in Washington's inner city as a response to the unmet needs of homeless people. People found out by word of mouth that they could receive health care with dignity and without waiting for long periods, as they often did in traditional outpatient departments and emergency rooms (Bargmann, 1985).

Although many health clinics have been developed in response to the needs of homeless people, they often also treat the domiciled poor, especially those who live in the immediate neighborhood. Other clinics were originally developed to serve poor people in general and now, for various reasons, find themselves serving increasing numbers of homeless people.

SPECIALIZED HEALTH CARE APPROACHES

Various other programs address the special needs of homeless people or the problems of specific subpopulations among the homeless.

Respite and Convalescent Care

One of the most serious issues facing those who work with homeless people is that many standard forms of treatment assume that the patient has a home; when that is not true, treatment is extraordinarily difficult. Convalescent (or respite) services allow a homeless person to recover from an illness or an injury that does not require (or no longer requires) care in a hospital but that is of such severity that the homeless person should not return to a regular shelter setting.

One example of a private effort is Christ House in Washington, D.C. As a result of a bequest, the Church of the Savior acquired and renovated an abandoned apartment house and converted it into a 34-bed respite facility; it has a paid and volunteer staff, including medical and nursing supervision and care. The Columbia Road Physician Group provides medical support, and all four doctors involved in the project live, with their families, on the top floor of the building, so that medical attention is available around the clock. When more intensive care is needed, local hospitals are used.

A similar program is the 40-bed respite unit at the Charles H. Gay Shelter Care Center for Men in New York City, which is a public–private effort. The shelter (including the respite unit) is funded by the New York City Human Resources Administration and is administered by the Volunteers of America, which is under contract with the city. The respite unit is adjacent to the on-site medical and nursing clinic administered by

St. Vincent's Hospital (see above) and receives nursing support from the clinic. Referral for backup hospital services is either to St. Vincent's Hospital or to one of the hospitals of the New York City Health and Hospitals Corporation.

Residential Placement

Many homeless people with physical disabilities, mental disabilities, or both who cannot live independently require supportive living settings. One program that attempts to meet this need is the Veterans Administration (VA) community placement program, which secures supervised housing for mentally or physically disabled veterans who are facing discharge from a VA medical center and who would be at extreme risk of becoming homeless. Members of the committee visited four such placement sites in Lexington, Kentucky. Three were private homes in which the individual homeowner contracted with the VA to accept patients from the medical center (the largest program accepted up to eight men) for supervised residential living. The fourth program was a personal care home licensed by the Commonwealth of Kentucky. The personal care home received clients from the state agencies serving the mentally ill and the mentally retarded, as well as from the VA medical center. This facility is larger (over 15 beds) and was specifically designed to serve a population in greater need of medical and nursing care. Although the residences were supervised and certified by government agencies, the actual funding for the individual veterans comes from their own VA benefits.

In each of the programs identified above, communication and coordination were accomplished by individualized approaches developed over a period of time with systems that were more or less unique to each city. The programs were primarily targeted to the homeless; funding and other resources ranged from the purely charitable to the wholly publicly funded. However, a comprehensive, cohesive system of services is lacking. Even those programs that had strong ties with a hospital did not network with programs that serve, for example, the mentally ill or substance abusers.

THE JOHNSON-PEW HEALTH CARE FOR THE HOMELESS PROJECTS

The most significant event to occur in the area of health care for homeless people in recent years was the creation of the Health Care for the Homeless grants, funded jointly by the Robert Wood Johnson Foundation of Princeton, New Jersey, and the Pew Memorial Trust of Philadelphia. In many respects, the creation of this joint program reflected the growth of the homeless problem and the fact that agencies that had historically been able to provide services to the homeless could no longer cope with their increasing numbers. The national Health Care for the Homeless program was developed to provide cities (applications were limited to the 50 largest cities in the United States) with an opportunity to make a significant impact on health care delivery to the homeless. On December 12, 1983, in a joint news release, the two foundations announced what was, in effect, the first attempt to address this problem on other than a local level. Cosponsored by the U.S. Conference of Mayors, the program guidelines required that cities forge a coalition of disparate groups of health care professionals and institutions, volunteer organizations, religious groups, public agencies, shelter providers, and members of the philanthropic community. This coalition was charged with developing a program to meet the health care needs of the homeless, improving their access to other supportive services and entitlements, and developing a strategy for continuing the program services after the termination of foundation funding:

As such coalitions strengthened and institutionalized their functions, it was hoped that they would become permanent structures for addressing the health and related needs of the homeless beyond the four year grant period. (Clark et al., 1985)

Of the 50 cities eligible for the program, 45 submitted grant applications; of these, 18 were funded under the national program and 1 city was funded under a special arrangement. A total of $25 million was allocated by the foundations, and each city received up to $1.4 million for use during a 4-year period.

One issue frequently raised as a result of the Johnson-Pew projects is whether it is necessary to develop separate health care systems for the domiciled and for the homeless. The answer to that question depends on the resources of an individual community and the willingness of existing health care systems to respond to the needs of homeless people. Even the most rigid system can, over a period of time, change to accommodate new programs; therefore, when it is necessary to develop parallel programs, it is frequently with the expectation that at some future time the newer program will be incorporated into existing programs. An especially good example of this is the incorporation of the Nashville Johnson-Pew project into the municipal health department.

Structure of the Johnson-Pew Projects

The 19 Johnson-Pew projects are distinctly different and highly idiosyncratic, and as such, they reflect the specific needs of the 19 cities in which they are located. The original request for proposal issued by the Johnson and Pew organizations required that all proposals be developed by a broad-based community coalition. Therefore, not one of the 19 programs was incorporated as a separate entity (although several are now in the process of seeking such incorporation). Each grantee needed to establish a system of governance and fiscal accountability, in effect, a fiduciary agent. The more common models provide for the funds to be authorized to an existing health care-related or social service-related agency (e.g., in New York City, the United Hospital Fund of New York; in Philadelphia, the Philadelphia Health Management Corporation) or to a charitable foundation (e.g., in San Francisco, the Episcopal Archdiocese of California; in San Antonio, the United Way). In two cities (Newark and Phoenix), the funds go directly to agencies of the municipal government. It is not yet possible to determine which funding methods are most effective.

In some of the projects, services are provided by staff who are employees of the project, with a single set of policies and procedures. Some programs rely on contracts with existing providers of health care services, to provide either specialized services (e.g, dental care) or general health care services to a specific geographic area (e.g., the New York City project has contracts with three existing health care agencies that provide services in different boroughs of the city). Staff are employees of the contract agency and are subject to the policies and salary schedules of that agency. Sometimes a mixture of direct and contracted services is provided. Certain services—such as case management—are provided directly by salaried staff, while other services—such as clinic operations— are provided by a contractor.

How services actually get to homeless people is probably the most varied (and creative) aspect of the Johnson-Pew projects. The methods of service delivery include mobile vans outfitted as clinics, mobile teams going to existing programs that serve homeless people (particularly shelters and soup kitchens), and central clinics located in areas where homeless people can be found in substantial numbers.

Common Elements of Health Care Programs for the Homeless

Although the Johnson-Pew projects are just past the midpoint in their 4-year grants, much has already been learned from these projects. As with the earlier models, there is no statistical basis to determine a program's success.* In the course of its review and after many discussions with service providers as well as the homeless people who receive care,

---

* However, the Social and Demographic Research Institute data derived from the client contact reports of the various projects do represent the first such diagnostic and utilization statistical data drawn from more than just a single local source; they also represent a potential base for future evaluations of program effectiveness.

the committee identified the common elements that follow as especially significant.

Holistic Approach

Rather than treating an isolated health problem without considering the person's social or environmental situation, these programs provide treatments that recognize the interaction between the illness and the state of being homeless. The nature and level of the individual's entitlement benefits, for example, whether they are sleeping in the streets or in a shelter, where they get food, and so on, are taken into consideration in developing a treatment approach.

Outreach

Health care is brought to areas where homeless people can be found. These targeted services can then serve as a conduit by which other services (including application and advocacy for entitlement benefits) are offered.

Empathetic Staff

Staff are aware of the attitudes that increase their effectiveness in working with the homeless population. In particular, staff recognize the exigencies of survival that impinge on the day-to-day activities of the homeless and the effects of those demands on the individual's health and health care.

Multidisciplinary Approach

Teams working with the homeless encompass a range of disciplines, including physicians, nurses, physician's assistants, nurse practitioners, and social workers. Given the range and severity of illnesses present among the homeless population, when volunteers are used (especially medical or nursing students), proper supervision is provided.

Case Management and Coordination of Services

One of the most critical elements in serving the homeless involves the coordination of patient treatment and the provision of access to other health care and social services with the aim of breaking the cycle of homelessness. The most frequent approach is to include social workers as part of the multidisciplinary team. This individual keeps in touch with service providers at other treatment sites to ensure that the homeless person follows through with the treatment plan.

Continuity

Homeless individuals have few other people to rely on, often leading them to be very distrustful of people in general. The continuity of the program staff helps to build trust. Changes in personnel or disruptions in schedules increase their wariness; conversely, seeing familiar faces (especially if they can be treated by the same people both at an outreach site and then again in a clinic setting) increases their cooperation.

Range of Health Care Services

The final element is that successful programs offer a broad range of services. For example, they make some provision for convalescent care, prenatal care, and treatment for alcohol problems. Access to services such as convalescent care on discharge helps to prevent unnecessary rehospitalization. Not all programs are able to provide this range of services directly; however, they do recognize the service gaps and try to fill them in by working with other service providers.

The Health Care for the Homeless projects in the cities of Milwaukee, Nashville, and Detroit illustrate some of the structured and programmatic elements developed by the several Johnson-Pew projects. In Milwaukee, the project is administered by the Coalition for Community Health Care, Inc., a nonprofit organization established in 1979 to advocate the health care of indigent people. The Milwaukee project chose to contract with social service agencies for the social service component of the project and with four medical facilities for health care services. The medical facilities provide pharmaceutical and medical supplies, as well as x rays and laboratory services. The county hospital provides optometry services and the local community health centers provide podiatry services. Dental care is provided by the community health centers. By using multiple health care facilities, the cost of those services and supplies that were not funded by the Johnson-Pew projects is more evenly distributed. The Milwaukee project uses mobile teams that go to sites at which homeless people receive other (nonmedical) services. Paraprofessional outreach workers approach homeless or alcoholic people on the streets and assist them in obtaining financial entitlements and then permanent housing. The progress of these people is then followed as they participate in support groups for substance abuse and maintenance on medication.

In Nashville, one of the smaller cities in the project and one with even fewer services for homeless people, the original grantee organization was the Council of Community Services, Inc., a social services coordinating agency. The project established a stationary clinic, the Downtown Clinic, which was initially located between the two major shelters for homeless people. Staffed mostly with midlevel practitioners, including a physician's assistant and a family nurse practitioner, the clinic also has a full-time medical director who is a National Health Service Corps doctor. Clients come to the clinic because of its proximity to where they are sheltered and because of word-of-mouth recommendations. The clinic itself is a traditional outpatient facility, including an x-ray suite, which enables the staff to provide diagnostic work immediately rather than referring the clients elsewhere. Besides the stationary clinic, there is outreach to homeless people on the streets, on the river bank, in the shelters, and at various service agencies. Since the project began, the Meharry Community Mental Health Center and the Tennessee Department of Mental Health and Mental Retardation have provided funding for two mental health care professionals to work with the Johnson-Pew project, primarily in outreach to homeless chronically mentally ill people on the streets. As indicated earlier, the Nashville project will continue after Johnson-Pew funding has run out through incorporation into the Metropolitan Nashville/ Davidson County Health Department, which has now succeeded the Council of Community Services as the grantee organization.

In Detroit, the Health Care for the Homeless project is administered by the United Community Services of Metropolitan Detroit. The project contracts for some of its services and provides other services directly. Three clinical and two administrative staff are on the project's payroll, while other staff are paid for through contracts: a part-time clinical nurse on contract with the Detroit Department of Public Health and one part-time physician and an administrative staff member on contract with the Wayne State University School of Medicine. In addition, the Detroit Department of Public Health has provided the project with two full-time staff members paid for by that department: a physician and the project director. The project has both mobile teams and a stationary clinic. The mobile teams visit eight different sites (shelters and soup kitchens) during the course of a week. If a client needs a more thorough workup, a referral is made to the clinic, which operates one morning per week. The clinic is located in space at the Detroit Receiving Hospital that was made available at no cost; the hospital also provides the clinic with much of its supplies. While the project purchases most of its own medical supplies and pharmaceuticals, x-ray services are provided free of charge by the Detroit Department of Public Health and Detroit Receiving Hospital. Optometric care is provided through a unique partnership: Clients are referred by the project to the Detroit Optometric Institute for eye examinations and, if necessary, for glasses. The Optometric Institute bills the Fort Street Presbyterian Church, a downtown church with a history of helping the homeless, at a reduced rate and the church pays for all the optometric services. Podiatric services are provided by the Detroit

Department of Public Health; emergency dental services are provided at no cost by the health department, while general dental care is provided by the dental school of the University of Detroit on a sliding scale basis. The project has received a grant from the state of Michigan to fund mental health care services. However, if the client is already known to one of the neighborhood mental health care centers, a referral is made to that center rather than attempting to provide direct services. In times of emergency or crisis, clients are referred to Detroit Receiving Hospital for inpatient admission.

The three programs described above use various funding and administrative mechanisms for the provision of specific services (e.g., a hospital for x-ray services, a dental school for dental services, and a mental health center for psychiatric services). Multiple administrative arrangements place a more serious burden on the role of case management than if those services were all under one roof and provided by one agency. For example, in Detroit the Johnson-Pew project provides case management to its clients. However, the success of case management depends on feedback from the staff of the facilities to which the Johnson-Pew team refers clients; such feedback is not always forthcoming. It should also be mentioned that the clients of these projects are, primarily, individual adults. The provision of such services to families presents a different set of problems.

The three project examples illustrate the point that success does not necessarily depend on the form of governance (whether it be by a not-for-profit board, as part of an existing health care or social service agency, or by an established charitable foundation), the manner of administration (whether by direct provision of services or by contracting with existing service providers), or the method of operation (a centralized clinic in an area where homeless people congregate or mobile teams going from one area of a city to another). In fact, these modes may or may not apply to other cities; structure and administration seem to be most effective when they reflect the individual characteristics of a specific city. What appears to be most significant are the presence of all—or at least most—of the seven common elements of health care programs for the homeless described above.

Issues Raised by the Johnson-Pew Project Models

Stationary Clinics or Mobile Teams

Each of these models has a somewhat different approach to providing health care services to homeless people. The common denominator, however, is a permanent outreach component. In some instances, a stable clinic site may be developed that has outreach workers, and in other cases the mobile teams go to places where the clients congregate for services.

Each of the different components of these models has strengths and weaknesses. For example, stationary clinics are able to provide more sophisticated technology (e.g., x-rays and electrocardiograms [ECGs]). On the other hand, such clinics might be viewed as too threatening for clients, especially if these individuals have had negative experiences with emergency rooms or clinics in the past. The informality of shelters and soup kitchens may be perceived as less threatening than an outpatient clinic; therefore, mobile teams may be in a better position to overcome such initial reluctance. Guests at these sites often ask for blood pressure checks or adhesive bandages as a means of testing the health care professionals. However, such sites do not usually provide ancillary services, such as ECGs. Many of these sites reach clients who would not otherwise have access to care; unfortunately, the sites are somewhat less stable: Soup kitchens may close down for a week or a month because of a lack of funding or to give volunteers a rest; there is sometimes difficulty finding space to set up a temporary clinic with access to running water; soup kitchens and meal programs are often open only for a brief period of time in the middle of the day or in the evening; and programs for the homeless sometimes close in April and do not reopen until November. Although there may be large numbers of guests, the patient flow and the abbreviated hours make it difficult for the efficient and effective use of staff.

Small Social Service Agencies or Large Health Care Facilities

Locating health care services in a social service agency may often mean that ancillary services or specialty clinic appointments must be negotiated on a case-by-case basis, which is a time-consuming procedure. Moreover physicians, nurse practitioners, and physician's assistants might find it professionally isolating to practice health care outside of a health care facility. Recently, a New York City mobile health team for the homeless was transferred administratively from a very small neighborhood health care center to a large teaching hospital. While the move did not affect to any substantial extent the provision of direct services to their clients (they continued to receive the same services at the same sites), it was welcomed by team members because of the additional supports that a large facility could provide.

Direct Provision of Services or Contracting Services

The model of contracting of services, while appropriate in many instances, may pose specific problems. If the contracted staff are employed by a major health care agency, they may experience a division of loyalties between their employer and the program that specifically serves the homeless. Such contract agencies often have different personnel policies in terms of holidays, vacations and pay scales, opportunities for advancement, staff development programs, and so on. These differences can negatively affect the morale of team members who work for different employers.

Size of Areas To Be Served

Another area of concern in developing models for delivering health care is the size of the geographic area to be served. In some Johnson-Pew cities, services have been focused in one downtown area where there may be the heaviest concentration of homeless people, effectively excluding large numbers of homeless people outside that catchment area. Other cities have tried to cover as broad an area as possible, which may result in the loss of valuable service delivery time because of the amount of time spent in transit. If the area covered is substantial, a sizable number of backup agreements may be necessary to ensure the provision of ancillary and diagnostic laboratory services for each treatment site. To a great extent, the combination or range of services and the geographic size of the area to be served are dependent on the amount of resources available.

TARGETED SERVICES FOR POPULATIONS WITH SPECIAL NEEDS

Concurrent with the development of the Johnson-Pew Health Care for the Homeless projects, other new forms of services to the homeless have been introduced. These programs provide health care to specific subpopulations among the homeless such as the chronically mentally ill, adolescents and youth, and homeless people with AIDS (acquired immune deficiency syndrome). Not only do they represent a growing recognition of the heterogeneity of the homeless population, they also indicate an increasing awareness that specific populations among the homeless require specific health care services designed to meet their particular needs.

The Chronically Mentally Ill*

Studies of the mental health of homeless people indicate that the prevalence of serious mental disorders is considerably higher among the homeless than it is among the general population (see Chapter 3). The

---

* This section is based in part on Breakey (in press) cited in Robertson and Greenbelt (in press).

provision of mental health services to homeless people is made difficult primarily by the lack of appropriate facilities and resources and by their extreme poverty, their lack of insight into their psychiatric problems, their distaste for psychiatric treatment, and the complexities of their service needs. Those needs, therefore, are often poorly met (Lamb, 1984).

As with homeless people in general, the seven elements delineated from the experience of the Johnson-Pew projects (a holistic approach, access and outreach, empathic staff, interdisciplinary approach, case management, continuity of services, and broad range of services) are also important in creating services for the homeless chronically mentally ill. To ensure effective treatment for this group, specialized forms of housing (including a range of supportive services, from independent living with minimal supervision to round-the-clock supervision in a community residence) and rehabilitation programs are also essential.

Housing

For severely mentally ill people, specialized housing arrangements are needed. In the wake of deinstitutionalization, various supervised housing arrangements have been developed. Model programs such as Fountain House in New York, a private, not-for-profit agency, combine a treatment center with supportive living in nearby apartments. With respect to public programs, one recent effort is the attempt of the New York State Office of Mental Health to provide supportive housing ranging in size from small community residences of fewer than 15 beds to the proposed larger residential care centers that resemble SRO hotels. Such centers, although funded by the state, are generally operated by well-established not-for-profit agencies. One of the requirements for funding is that the sponsoring agency must guarantee the provision of full-day treatment services for all residents of the facility, either directly or by means of contracts with other agencies. In addition, for those individuals whose disabilities are so severe as to warrant it, such services must be provided on-site until such time as the individual is able to negotiate community systems.

Rehabilitation

Structured psychosocial rehabilitation programs are often necessary to enable mentally ill people to function at their maximum capacity in the community. For the homeless, in most cases, the very structure of such programs may be a deterrent. Therefore, the principles of psychosocial rehabilitation must be brought to the shelters or residences. Over time, this should enable the individual to move from the on-site setting to a community setting. Assistance is also needed for homeless people to regain lost skills in the activities of daily living (ADL) that most of us take for granted (e.g., personal hygiene, cleaning, and basic meal preparation). The Community Support Systems program at the Volunteers of America shelter in New York is an example of such an effort. It provides a model apartment as part of an ADL skills training program. A similar program exists in Phoenix, where six apartments are used to help chronically mentally ill homeless people learn the skills required for independent living before moving into such situations.

A comprehensive array of services is needed by chronically mentally ill homeless people, but in most communities a full range of services does not exist. Until comprehensive service systems for mentally ill homeless people are developed, the care that clinicians can give to these patients is limited.

The committee and staff visited several programs for the homeless mentally ill. In addition to serving as potential models for services to chronically mentally ill homeless people, they are also possible solutions to the problems of other subpopulations. Some of these programs are described below.

Robert Wood Johnson Foundation Project for the Chronically Mentally Ill

The original Johnson-Pew Health Care for the Homeless program did not include specific services for homeless people who are mentally ill. Subsequently, the Robert Wood Johnson Foundation initiated a program to address the issue of providing services to the chronically mentally ill (including the homeless) in early 1986. It is jointly sponsored by the U.S. Conference of Mayors and by the U.S. Department of Housing and Urban Development, which has committed $75 million in additional support for Section 8 housing certificates. This program, administered by the Department of Psychiatry of Harvard Medical School, seeks to develop systems of coordinated services to the chronically mentally ill in the nine cities that receive funding under its auspices. The program attempts to bring disparate funding and organizational systems into a unified structure, so that the chronically mentally ill person need not go from place to place to receive services and run the risk of neglect. In addition, the housing component is designed to support the clinical component by providing housing appropriate to the individual's level of disability.

Self-Help Centers

During their site visit to the San Francisco area, several committee members toured the Oakland Independence Support Center. This is a day treatment center for homeless mentally ill people that is operated and staffed exclusively by people who themselves have been treated (either as inpatients or as outpatients) for mental illness. The center is run on the basis of group decisions regarding programs and has proved to be especially effective in obtaining housing for its "members," primarily because it is willing to assist both the tenant and the landlord in resolving problems and disputes. Because of this willingness to maintain extensive involvement with members and to intervene to resolve such problems, landlords tend to seek out people involved with the center as tenants. Similar self-help centers have been developed in other cities. Self-help centers such as this one are partly dependent on the leadership of an individual or a small group.

Outreach Street Teams

A third approach for providing services to the homeless mentally ill is the development of outreach teams specifically seeking to identify homeless people in need of services. As indicated before, the Nashville Johnson-Pew Health Care for the Homeless (HCH) project has been supplemented by funding from the Tennessee Department of Mental Health and Mental Retardation's community initiative program that provides two case managers to walk the streets, developing rapport with chronically mentally ill homeless people. A similar effort is directly funded by the Johnson-Pew project in Los Angeles; there, the outreach worker was himself once a homeless person. The Volunteers of America (VOA) outreach program at transportation facilities of the Port Authority of New York and New Jersey also makes extensive use of former homeless people as members of their teams. The VOA program is jointly funded by an interstate compact agency and by a department of the local government (the New York City Department of Mental Health). New York is also the site of one of the most highly publicized programs, Project Reachout, which sends staff into Central Park to make contact with homeless people who literally live in the park (Goddard-Riverside Community Centers, 1986).

Veterans Administration Homeless Chronically Mentally Ill Program

One of the most recent and most extensive efforts to address the needs of the mentally ill homeless is the Homeless Chronically Mentally Ill (HCMI) program operated by the VA as mandated by P.L. 100-6. The law was enacted on February 12, 1987, and the program was operational within 4 months, an accomplishment made even more notable by the fact that this program encompasses 43 sites in 26 states. In its first 4 months of operation (May to September 1987), the outreach staff made contact with 6,342 homeless veterans. In designing the program, the staff of the VA's Division of Mental Health and Behavioral Sciences made extensive use of the experience of some of the programs previously described in this chapter, especially the Johnson-Pew HCH projects* (Rosenheck et al., 1987).

Briefly, the program is operated out of 43 (of the 172) VA medical centers throughout the country. Outreach teams of two or more staff work in the streets and at community sites (e.g., shelters and soup kitchens) at which homeless people congregate; the HCMI staff identified such unusual points of contact as the middle of a sandbar in a river in Oregon and under a bridge in Indianapolis. Of the total number of contacts made, 64 percent took place in the community, 30.2 percent at VA medical centers, and 3.5 percent at veteran centers; 61 percent of the contacts were initiated by HCMI staff, 17 percent by the veterans, and 12 percent by referral from community-based programs.

The basic structure of the program is as follows: outreach contact, intake assessment, psychiatric and medical assessments, linkage with existing providers of services (both VA and non-VA), residential treatment if necessary, and comprehensive community-based mental health treatment if necessary. As is often the case with such programs, there is a steady drop in numbers as homeless people move through such a process. Of the 6,342 homeless people with whom contact was made during the first 4 months of the program, only 4,010 completed the intake assessment phase; of those, only one-third completed the psychiatric assessment and only one-fifth completed the medical assessment. This can be attributed in part to the fact that the psychiatric and medical assessments were performed primarily at VA medical centers (sites to which many homeless veterans are wary of going); the VA reports that it is actively pursuing alternate sites in the community. Despite these problems, the VA reported 360 placements in residential treatment during the same period.

The VA HCMI program has several features worth noting. First, early in the program the decision was made to include those "at serious risk" of homelessness among those who would be eligible for services. Of those veterans for whom an intake assessment was completed, 8.7 percent were in intermittent residence with family or friends and 8.5 percent had a room or apartment of their own from which they were in danger of eviction. This makes the HCMI programs one of the few such programs to address formally the issue of preventing homelessness.

---

* For a full description of the HCMI program, see Rosenheck et al. (1987). For a brief description of the veterans seen in this program, see Chapter 1 of this report.

Second, due to the relatively isolated location of many of the 43 VA medical centers included in the program, the VA made a policy decision to contract with non-VA programs to provide residential treatment at sites near where the homeless veterans are found. In addition, provision has been made to offer community-oriented case management during and after such treatment to stabilize such placements.

Finally, prior to start-up and continuing through implementation, the VA provided training to the outreach workers, first at four regional training sessions conducted in Alabama, California, Missouri, and Virginia. This training involved such sophisticated techniques as videotaped demonstrations and role playing. Subsequent follow-up included site visits by staff from the VA central office in Washington, D.C., to staff in the field and monthly telephone conference calls with staff at all 43 sites.

Alcohol and Drug Abuse

As with the mentally ill, a homeless person who is an alcohol abuser is unlikely to benefit from an approach that does not include a range of services. Nonalcohol substance abuse is a more recent phenomenon and appears to be limited somewhat to younger homeless people (under age 40) and to certain cities, primarily on the East Coast. Again, this population needs a full range of services, including specialized housing. The committee was able to identify several programs targeted toward homeless people with alcohol or drug problems. The Guest House in Milwaukee serves a homeless population that is evenly divided between the chronically mentally ill and chronic substance abusers. Harbor House in St. Louis is an alcohol rehabilitation program for homeless men; health care services are provided to Harbor House by a local voluntary hospital.

The following are some examples of programs that have been described in the professional literature.

• Case management teams, such as those funded by the Illinois Department of Alcoholism and Substance Abuse.

• Shelters specifically for homeless people who are alcoholics or drug abusers; the Illinois Department of Alcoholism and Substance Abuse funds three such programs, as does the Massachusetts Division of Alcoholism and Drug Rehabilitation. The Maine Office of Alcoholism and Drug Abuse Prevention funds four shelters, one of which is also the site of a bakery that is used to provide training and employment for the homeless clients.

• Programs for permanent or long-term housing, such as those funded by the Massachusetts Division of Alcoholism and Drug Rehabilitation; alcohol-free housing programs developed in Los Angeles, Seattle, and Portland, Oregon. In addition,

• Intensive residential programs that combine treatment on-site; one example of this is a program in New Jersey, funded by the state Division of Alcoholism. Under this program, a small (10-person) group home for homeless alcoholics is also the setting for day activities (e.g., counseling, vocational training, education, and leisure time activities), as well as referrals for health and mental health care services.

These examples indicate that programs can be developed to address the needs of homeless people who have problems with alcohol or drugs.

AIDS

It has been only 8 years since AIDS was first publicly identified. Since then the disease has reached epidemic proportions, and services for people that have been affected have not kept pace with demand. This is especially true for homeless people with AIDS. During a site visit to San Francisco, members of the committee met with the AIDS Advisory Committee of the San Francisco City/County Department of Public Health, as well as the AIDS discrimination specialist of the San Francisco Human Rights Commission. That meeting basically confirmed that those issues described in the Institute of Public Services Performance, Inc., report in New York (see Chapter 2) are not limited to any one community. The advisory committee reported that such matters as loss of housing due to loss of employment, discrimination, or while awaiting entitlement eligibility determinations are very real problems.

Members of the committee toured the Folsom Street Hotel program in San Francisco, a residential program for homeless people with AIDS operated by Catholic Charities, with partial funding by the City and County of San Francisco. Although it did not tour the facility, the committee is also aware of Bailey House, a similar program in New York City that is operated by the AIDS Resource Center with funding from the New York City Human Resources Administration and a grant from the U.S. Department of Health and Human Services. Both of these programs were developed to provide housing and supportive services to this population. However, because many patients with AIDS are increasingly disabled as the disease progresses, additional forms of housing with varying levels of physical care, up to and including skilled nursing facilities and hospices, are needed. The alternative seems to be hospitalization, which is extremely expensive.

Homeless Individual Women, Families, and Youths

Adult Individual Women

Other subpopulations among the homeless have been identified in recent years as needing specific targeted approaches. Members of the committee toured several programs for homeless individual adult women. Site visits were conducted to the House of Ruth, a shelter for homeless women in Washington, D.C., and the Firehouse Annex, a drop-in center and transitional residence for homeless women in Chicago. While neither of these programs is specifically a health care program, both are clinic sites for their respective city's Johnson-Pew HCH projects. Another issue in evaluating services for homeless women is the high reported prevalence of mental illness among them. The committee toured a program for homeless emotionally disturbed women at the YWCA in San Diego, a program funded in part by the San Diego County Division of Mental Health Services.

Families

The committee visited programs for homeless families in several cities, in particular Pilgrim House in Kansas City and Project Hope in Boston. These two programs are not specifically health care programs; however, Pilgrim House receives on-site health care services from Kansas City's mobile homeless health care team, and Project Hope receives services from the Boston Johnson-Pew family team. Another program that the committee toured was the Emergency Lodge in St. Louis, a large shelter for homeless families operated by the Salvation Army. Among the services provided to the families are daily health screening sessions and health education programs conducted by a public health nurse and a weekly clinic conducted by a volunteer health screening team. This program is unique in that it also has a free day care center, which enables homeless mothers to search for jobs during the day.

One program that specifically addresses the health care needs of homeless families is the Venice Family Clinic in Los Angeles. This is a free clinic that has been serving the Venice Beach/Santa Monica area for more than 17 years; its program has been augmented by the Los Angeles Johnson-Pew project to allow for services to homeless families. St. Anthony's Clinic in San Francisco, operated by the St. Anthony Foundation, serves both homeless families and homeless individual adult men; however, in response to fears expressed by homeless mothers about single men, the clinic has separate entrances and treatment suites for each group. Although these two programs certainly are excellent examples of what can be done, actual programs specifically serving homeless families do not exist anywhere in the numbers needed, especially in light of reports that this is the fastest growing subpopulation among the homeless.

Homeless Youths

The three studies of homeless youths cited in Chapter 1 (Boston, New York, and Toronto) each reported on shelter populations. Despite the differences among the study populations, the similarities in the findings regarding the physical and mental health needs of this population are even more significant. All three studies reported that supportive services, rather than the provision of housing alone, are needed. Each also reported that both the number of attempts to run away and the length of time that the teenager has been away or in shelter(s) are important. The greater the number of attempts to run away and the longer the adolescent is in an institutional setting, the more difficult it becomes to place that youth in a noninstitutional setting or, having made such a placement, for that youth to remain there. While the three studies disagreed on the form that noninstitutional services should take, they agreed that, given the problems of this population, specialized services for this group are necessary.

The study by the Greater Boston Adolescent Emergency Network (1985) of Massachusetts emphasized the changing role of shelters in the network of youth services.

In the 1960s and 70s a network of emergency shelters was developed across the country to house an increasing number of "true runaways," young teens who had fled from a horrific home environment and had no place to sleep. From the phone booth on the corner or from a poster on a bus station wall, they were able to locate the nearest shelter and find a safe haven. Today, this still happens, but it is the exception, not the rule. . . . Due to the lack of other resources to accommodate and treat the chronic system youth, emergency shelters have become 30 to 45 day warehouses for adolescents with no place to go. Twenty percent (20%) of our sample were referred to shelter care not to manage a crisis, but specifically to shelter the youth while long-term care was being arranged. An additional 15 percent were referred from another temporary shelter.

Members of the committee toured the Larkin Street Youth Center in San Francisco. This program, funded in part by federal, state, and local governments and in part by charitable donations, serves runaway and throwaway youths in the Tenderloin section of that city. It provides services, including health and mental health care services, in a drop-in setting. The center reports a 74 percent success rate in getting youths off the streets; of those youths that have been helped, 40 percent have been returned to their families and 60 percent have been placed in foster care, usually in the communities from which they originally came. The center also has a very strong AIDS education program, a critical issue because so many of the adolescents have become involved with intravenous drug abuse, prostitution, or both.

In addition to the common element of being aimed toward specific subpopulations, many of these programs also exist as a result of joint public and private support. Some, such as the Nashville outreach program and the San Diego YWCA program, receive support from their state mental health agencies. Others, like Bailey House in New York and the

Folsom Street Hotel program in San Francisco, receive funding from municipal agencies. Still others, such as the Medeiros Center in Boston, receive funding from specific federal programs. Finally, some programs, such as the Larkin Street Youth Center in San Francisco, receive funding from several levels of government or, as is the case with the Volunteers of America outreach program in New York City, from specialized public authorities. What is noteworthy is that in each case additional resources have been forthcoming from the charitable sector, representing a true public and private cooperation.

OTHER ISSUES IN HEALTH SERVICES FOR THE HOMELESS

Coordinated Efforts in Non-Johnson-Pew Cities

In addition to inquiring into cities that have received grants from the Johnson-Pew Health Care for the Homeless project, the committee sought information as to how health and mental health care is being provided to the homeless in cities that did not receive such grants. Site visits were made to three cities that applied for the grants but that were not funded (Kansas City, St. Louis, and San Diego) and one city that, because it was not among the 50 largest, was not eligible (Lexington, Kentucky). Returning to the four elements that appear to be common throughout most programs providing treatment to the homeless, the committee was able to make several observations.

Communication

Notwithstanding the lack of specific funding for health care programs for the homeless, each of the four cities evidenced effective communication networks. Even though Kansas City and St. Louis were not successful applicants for the grant funding, the coalitions that were developed during the preparation of their applications continue in existence. This enabled the process of communication developed for the grant proposal to proceed further; each city chose to attempt (with some success) to implement the original grant proposal with other sources of funding. In San Diego there have been several successive coalitions and task forces that have enabled communication networks to expand, often with the city and the county governments taking an active role. In Lexington, which was not eligible to apply for a grant and therefore did not specifically need a broad-based coalition for this purpose, such a coalition exists nonetheless because of close cooperation among provider agencies and a very supportive municipal government.

Coordination

Partly because they decided to proceed along the lines of their original grant proposals, Kansas City and St. Louis have achieved a reasonable level of coordination of services. In Lexington, in part because of its small size (population of approximately one-half million), coordination is less formal, but no less effective. San Diego, on the other hand, faces a serious problem arising from a separation of areas of responsibility mandated by the state of California: the county has responsibility for health care, mental health care, and social services and the city has responsibility for housing and public safety. Although the Johnson-Pew grant has enabled two other California cities (Los Angeles and San Francisco) to overcome this problem to some extent (especially in San Francisco, which has a combined city and county government), San Diego still faces serious problems of coordination of services.

Targeted Approaches

Each of these cities attempted to develop targeted services, especially health care services. Lexington has placed services for the homeless in one area in the downtown section of the city. St. Louis has residential programs near the psychiatric hospital that serves many chronically mentally ill homeless people. Kansas City is currently attempting to target services to homeless families, a problem that appears to be exacerbated by the economic decline of the surrounding farm communities. The San Diego County Department of Health Services has recently provided some funding for a clinic operated in the downtown area in which homeless people tend to congregate. None of these cities, however, has been able to develop the kind of specialized services that are provided by many of the Johnson-Pew projects.

Funding

In three of these four cities, attempts to provide health care services to homeless people have been with joint public and private funding, with the bulk of the public funding coming from the city governments. In San Diego, however, the health care programs are mandated to the county government, with the result that program locations are distant from the areas where homeless people are found, transportation is difficult to obtain, and it is time-consuming to travel to the programs; these are serious barriers to access.

The experiences of these four cities support the fact that specific efforts are needed to deliver health care services to the homeless and to earmark funds for such efforts. Even where programs do exist for homeless people, the lack of access and the absence of a targeted effort may vitiate them.

Range of Health Care Services

The experience of the Johnson-Pew projects and other providers of health care services for homeless people suggests that a wide range of services is needed. The range and the extent to which each service should be developed in a given city may be based upon such factors as the numbers of homeless people and the proportions of the various homeless subpopulations. An assumption of these health care services is that provision of social services is an integral component of health care.

Although many of these services are appropriate for all people (homeless or not) and are especially important for the medically indigent, they are of even greater importance to homeless people because of the high level of debilitation seen in that population. The following range of services could be considered basic primary health care for homeless people.

1. Outreach to people where they are, including the streets.
2. General medical assessment and treatment for chronic and acute illnesses.
3. Specific screening, treatment, and follow-up for such health problems as high blood pressure.
4. Pediatric services (including well-baby clinics, immunizations, and screening for lead poisoning) and diagnostic and psychosocial intervention programs for both preschool and school-age children to address emotional disability and developmental delays.
5. Ancillary services (dentistry, podiatry, optometry, and specialized diets).
6. Access to mental health care and substance abuse services, including access to specialized housing.
7. Referral and access to convalescent care, as well as long-term medical and nursing care for catastrophic illness.
8. Gynecological services.
9. Prenatal care.
10. Educational services, primarily with regard to family planning and the prevention of sexually transmitted diseases (including the free distribution of condoms as part of AIDS education efforts).

Any health care providers also should take into consideration specialized mental health and substance abuse services. Unfortunately, health, mental health, and substance abuse have traditionally had separate funding streams, even though all three can interact with each other. This often blocks the delivery of services to people with multiple diagnoses. Models for the treatment of dual or multiple diagnoses for homeless people are rare (the Prevention Research Center in Berkeley, California, is currently researching the limited models of services for homeless substance abusers). The fact that they do not exist in great numbers does not, however, indicate that there is not a great need for such services; all reports received (both from the literature and from the site visits) suggest just the opposite.

Discharge Planning

Discharge planning is a difficult and complex task at best. General hospitals, mental hospitals, mental retardation facilities, correctional facilities, and the foster care system often are remote from the community into which the person is being discharged. However, all of these service providers are mandated to develop discharge plans for each client or patient, and even the best of plans can break down. Often, there is no follow-up to determine whether the plan works, and there can be an almost total lack of communication and coordination among institutions, communities, and the income support and service systems. The core of the problem, however, is that there are not enough options available on discharge. Acute-care hospitals are discharging people earlier, and homeless people have no adequate place to recuperate. There are only a few facilities that are minimally comparable to Christ House in Washington, D.C., and one cannot discharge a homeless person to home care if there is no home. It is true that there are insufficient appropriate options for discharging homeless people from acute-care hospitals; but networks of institutional providers, community-based service providers for the homeless, and the public social welfare offices could at least facilitate a more appropriate discharge than to the streets or to an inappropriate shelter. It is also highly desirable that shelter providers set aside beds that could be used for infirmary care or convalescence.

Similarly, mental health programs could plan for discharging homeless people to a supportive living residence with an appropriate level of care. The short supply of such programs makes it difficult to develop discharge plans, but more extensive planning before and follow-up after discharge might prevent a significant number of failed placements. Correctional facilities and parole officers could better coordinate and monitor more intensively an individual immediately following discharge, when that person is most likely to be unemployed and is at a higher risk of becoming homeless. As noted previously, however, the lack of a full range of community-based placements is the worst problem in discharge planning, so that clients, patients, or ex-prisoners are thwarted from achieving the most independent level of functioning of which they are capable.

One seemingly critical issue relates to the preparations for the discharge of an individual who may be eligible for Supplemental Security Income benefits. Although it is not adequately publicized, the Social Security Administration does have a program for early predischarge application and review, primarily directed to those in psychiatric inpatient facilities (U.S. Congress, House, Committee on Ways and Means, 1987). Every effort should be made to utilize this program so that disabled people who might be eligible for SSI could conceivably have the application approved concurrently with their discharge. Unfortunately, the Social Security Administration does not yet have a procedure for early application and review.

Case Management

Over the course of this study, the committee heard repeated references to case management. During its site visits, the committee met and spoke with a number of individuals identified as case managers. These people came from a wide variety of backgrounds, including social work, psychology, nursing, and in one instance, from the ranks of the homeless themselves.

How one views case management often seems to depend on the viewer's own past experience with the case management process, both personal and professional. Some see case management as the critical link that determines the success or failure of a program. Others see case managers as just another level of organizational bureaucracy that serves as still another barrier to the access of services.

The major problem appears to be that case management is ill defined and the role of the case manager is inadequately described. Fortunately, during the course of this study two publications were released that sought— from very different approaches—to resolve this problem. The Task Force on Welfare Prevention of the National Governors' Association (NGA) has released a report (1987) on welfare reform, *Productive People, Productive Policies,* that views the role of case management and case managers in terms of all human services. The COSMOS Corporation, under contract with the National Institute of Mental Health, has published a report, *Intensive Case Management for Persons Who Are Homeless and Mentally Ill* (Andranovich and Rosenblum, 1987). These two reports together provide a wealth of information for anyone who wishes to read a detailed analysis of this process and for those who work with homeless people.

The COSMOS report presents the following definition of case management:

Case management, as a mechanism for facilitating the access and movement of an individual through fragmented service systems, is viewed as an essential feature for effective service delivery to individuals who are homeless and seriously mentally ill. It attempts to ensure that a community support system is maximally responsive to the specific, multiple, and changing needs of individual clients.

Both the NGA and the COSMOS reports identify similar functions that constitute the structure of case management:

- *identification and outreach*—determining who is in need of services and bringing them into the service delivery system;
- *assessment*—determining the client's individual strengths and determining the needs that must be met;
- *service planning*—developing a plan to meet those needs;
- *coordination and facilitation*—working with the client and service providers to arrange for the actual delivery of services necessary to meet those needs;
- *monitoring*—working with the client and service providers to determine whether each service provider (or all service providers, if there is more than one) is meeting its obligations;
- *evaluating*—determining when and if changes in the service delivery plan are necessary and then negotiating and monitoring the implementation of those changes; and
- *advocacy*—acting for or with the client in obtaining those services (including housing) that are needed, with one of the ultimate goals being that the client eventually becomes his or her own advocate.

The COSMOS report also identified "intensive" case management as critical to working with chronically mentally ill homeless people. It defined intensive case management as a more aggressive approach for those most in need, especially in the areas of outreach and advocacy. In addition, the NGA report speaks to the need for certain qualities in those who are case managers:

- communication skills, both with the client and with service providers;
- knowledge of such things as rules, regulations, programs, and resources;
- empathy with the client and the ability to assist in seeing the client's strengths and to capitalize on those strengths;
- ability to identify the critical issues facing the client and to identify the appropriate resolutions for those issues; and
- ability to hold others—both the client and the service providers—accountable for their performance.

Liability Insurance Coverage for Providers

The committee received several reports of programs that have encountered difficulties in obtaining malpractice insurance. Part of the problem may be that the programs are based in social service agencies rather than in health care facilities, but the committee is unaware of instances in which legal judgments have been rendered in favor of a homeless plaintiff in a malpractice action. Therefore, the basis for setting extraordinarily high premiums for or denying malpractice insurance is unclear. The committee also received reports that several not-for-profit organizations lost their liability insurance coverage or were charged very high premiums, causing them to either suspend or curtail operations for extended periods of time. At present, these reports appear to be scattered and do not seem to represent any specific pattern of denial of coverage. The potential negative impact of the loss of insurance coverage on the ability of the private sector to continue to provide services to homeless people cannot be ignored.

The potential lack of insurance coverage is of special concern with respect to the growing involvement of universities (especially medical, dental, and nursing schools) in the provision of health care services to the homeless. The committee observed the involvement of the schools of nursing of the University of Kentucky in the programs for the homeless in Lexington and of the University of California, Los Angeles, in the Johnson-Pew project in Los Angeles. In addition, the committee is aware of similar programs with the Johns Hopkins Medical Institutions in Baltimore and the Georgetown University Dental School in Washington, D.C. Problems with insurance—both malpractice and general liability—could effectively forestall such efforts.

Personnel

Staff recruited to work with homeless people often have some special characteristics as well as professional expertise: They are willing to work against all kinds of odds and to provide services where the people are, leaving behind the more traditional and protected clinic and office settings. The ability to be innovative and flexible is important for working with the homeless. Staff may be open to the development of techniques that are different from those of the academic medical model and the usual adult outpatient clinics. The treatment of health problems is complicated by all the psychosocial problems experienced by homeless individuals and families. Some clients may be distrustful, rejecting, or hostile. The problems presented may often overwhelm the best trained, most experienced workers. Many of the adaptive, creative responses that homeless people develop for coping on the street may work against their being moved into a domiciled situation. Making such changes and adaptations may be overwhelming and frightening for homeless people to contemplate. Finding the innovative approach to engaging such clients and motivating them to try changes is the ultimate challenge of professionals who work with homeless people.

Of central importance to the task is each staff member's commitment and willingness to work as a part of an interdisciplinary team in which there is distinct professional expertise but also some fluidity in roles. In addition, although it is unlikely that anyone would be attracted to working with homeless people for material reasons, too often the salaries that are offered reflect society's tendency to stigmatize the workers in the same manner as it stigmatizes homeless people. Salaries can be made commensurate with work load and experience as well as competitive in the employment market. Specific and appropriate training of staff is desirable. Some staff may already have worked with homeless people but not in the context of health care services; others may be health care workers who have not worked with homeless people. Still others may have worked with a different population of homeless individuals. Training might include:

- issues relating to the homeless, for example, the causes of homelessness, the subpopulations, and the health problems of homeless people;
- orientation to the agency, including its policies, procedures, and opportunities for staff development;
- supervision, including the medical and social service aspects of the program;
- interview techniques or other means of assessing emotional problems;
- crisis intervention techniques;
- problems of working with the chronically mentally ill;
- identification of and strategies for confronting manipulative behaviors; and
- issues of case management, for example, other resources that are available and how a homeless person can access those resources.

SUMMARY

Although homeless people are a diverse group, the nature of their life situations and the multiplicity of their needs lead to the conclusion that they would benefit from specific approaches in the provision of health and mental health care services. Programs have been targeted to the homeless in general; specific programs have been targeted to certain subpopulations that are delineated by the nature of their health problems, demographic characteristics that necessitate specialized approaches, or their location, such as in rural and suburban areas. Even when such specialized services are provided, the coordination of efforts with other existing services is essential. The goal should be to enable homeless people to have access to the range of services that already exist, thereby decreasing their need for specialized services. The ultimate goal is to resolve whatever problems prevent homeless people from becoming domiciled.

REFERENCES

Andranovich, G. D., and S. Rosenblum. 1987. Intensive Case Management for Persons Who Are Homeless and Mentally Ill. Washington, D.C.: COSMOS Corporation.

Bargmann, E. 1985. Washington, D.C.: The Zacchaeus Clinic—A model of health care for homeless people. In Health Care of Homeless People, P. W. Brickner, L. K. Scharer, B. Conanan, A. Elvy, and M. Savarese, eds. New York: Springer-Verlag.

Breakey, W. R. In press. Mental Health Services for Homeless People. In Homelessness: A National Perspective. M. Robertson and M. Greenblatt, eds. New York: Plenum.

Brickner, P. W., L. K. Scharer, B. Conanan, A. Elvy, and M. Savarese, eds. 1985. Health Care of Homeless People. New York: Springer-Verlag.

Clark, M. E., R. M. Neal, S. L. Neibacher, and S. L. Wobido. 1985. A flexible approach to health services for the homeless: The National Health Care for the Homeless Program. Paper presented at the Annual Meeting of the American Public Health Association, Washington, D.C.

Fischer, P. J., and W. R. Breakey. 1986. Characteristics of the homeless with alcohol problems in Baltimore: Some preliminary results. Department of Health Policy and Management, School of Hygiene and Public Health, and Department of Psychiatry and Behavioral Sciences, School of Medicine, The Johns Hopkins University, Baltimore, Md.

Goddard-Riverside Community Centers. 1986. Project Reachout: Services and Advocacy for the Mentally Ill Homeless. New York: Goddard-Riverside Community Centers.

Greater Boston Adolescent Emergency Network. 1985. Ride a Painted Pony on a Spinning Wheel Ride. Boston: Massachusetts Committee for Children and Youth, Inc.

Lamb, H. R., ed. 1984. The Homeless Mentally Ill. Washington, D.C.: American Psychiatric Association.

Robertson, M., and M. Greenblatt. In press. Homelessness: The National Perspective. New York: Plenum.

Rosenheck, R., P. Gallup, C. Leda, P. Leaf, R. Milstein, I. Voynick, P. Errera, L. Lehman, G. Koerber, and R. Murphy. 1987. Progress Report on the Veterans Administration Program for Homeless Chronically Mentally Ill Veterans. Washington, D.C.: Veterans Administration.

Task Force on Welfare Prevention, National Governors' Association. 1987. Productive People, Productive Policies. Washington, D.C.: National Governors' Association.

U.S. Congress, House, Committee on Ways and Means. 1987. Background material and data on programs within the jurisdiction of the Committee on Ways and Means. 100th Cong., 1st sess., March 6, 1987.

6 Summary and Recommendations

ORIGIN OF THIS STUDY

Among congressional actions taken in recent years to address both the broader aspects of homelessness and the more narrow issues relating to the health of homeless people was the Health Professions Training Act of 1985 (P.L. 99-129). This mandated that the secretary of the Department of Health and Human Services ask the Institute of Medicine of the National Academy of Sciences to study the delivery of health care services to homeless people. This report is the result of that study.

The study committee was composed of experts in fields such as medicine, nursing, and social sciences; two public officials who administer statewide health and human services programs also served on the committee.

The charge to the committee and its staff was stated in P.L. 99-129:

1. evaluate whether existing eligibility requirements for health care services actually prevent homeless people from receiving those services;
2. evaluate the efficiency of health care services to homeless people; and
3. make recommendations as to what should be done by the federal, state, and local governments as well as private organizations to improve the availability and delivery of health care services to homeless people.

The members of the study committee endorse the analyses and conclusions of the report but unanimously wish to express their strong feeling that the recommendations are too limited in addressing the broader issues of homelessness—especially the supply of low-income housing, income maintenance, the availability of support services, and access to health care for the poor and uninsured.

At the request of the study's funding agency in the Department of Health and Human Services, the Health Resources and Services Administration, the committee took a broad view of health care and of needs for health care-related services, including matters such as nutrition, mental health, alcohol and drug abuse problems, and dental care.

STUDY PROCESS

The study committee met five times during a 10-month period (December 1986 to September 1987); individual committee members participated in site visits to 11 cities and to rural areas of four states to observe the problems of the homeless firsthand. The committee also commissioned 10 papers on specific areas of concern, such as the legal aspects of access to health care and the problems of providing health care for homeless people in the rural areas of America. Committee members, assisted by a study staff of two professionals, reviewed what is known about the health of homeless people, as evidenced in the scholarly literature, reports of public and private organizations, and—in particular—the ongoing evaluation of work of the 19 Health Care for the Homeless projects funded by the Robert Wood Johnson Foundation and the Pew Memorial Trust.

In the course of this study, the committee encountered several major methodological problems. For example, the lack of a uniform definition of homelessness results in substantial disagreement about the size of the homeless population. Some people define the homeless as only those who are on the streets or in shelters; others include those who are temporarily living with family or friends because they cannot afford housing. For its working definition, the committee adopted the one contained in the Stewart B. McKinney Homeless Assistance Act of 1987 (P.L. 100-77), which defines a homeless person as one who lacks a fixed, permanent nighttime residence or whose nighttime residence is a temporary shelter, welfare hotel, transitional housing for the mentally ill, or any public or private place not designed as sleeping accommodations for human beings (U.S. Congress, House, 1987).

The committee commissioned a study of the methodology of counting the homeless, which is included as Appendix B to this report, but refrained from providing its own quantitative estimate of the number of homeless people. One recent estimate of the number of homeless people in the United States, published in June 1988 by the National Alliance to End Homelessness (Alliance Housing Council, 1988), calculates that currently, on any given night, there are 735,000 homeless people in the United States; that during the course of 1988, 1.3 million to 2.0 million people will be homeless for one night or more; and that these people are among the approximately 6 million Americans who, because of their disproportionately high expenditures for housing costs, are at extreme risk of becoming homeless.

WHAT WAS LEARNED

Who Are the Homeless?

Contrary to the traditional stereotypes of homeless people, the homeless of the 1980s are not all single, middle-aged, male alcoholics. Neither are they all mentally ill people made homeless as a by-product of the policy of deinstitutionalization of mental health care.

The homeless are younger, more ethnically diverse, and increasingly are more likely to be members of families than is generally believed by the public. In most cities around the country, minorities—especially blacks and Hispanics—are represented disproportionately among the homeless as compared with their percentage of the overall population of those cities. Children under the age of 18, usually as part of a family headed by a mother, are the fastest growing group among the many subpopulations of the homeless. On the other hand, the elderly are underrepresented among the homeless in comparison with their percentage in the general population. There are a substantial number of veterans among the homeless, especially from the Vietnam era.

Homeless people tend to be long-term residents of the city in which they live. The homeless in rural areas, as well as homeless urban families, usually have gone through several stages of doubling up with family and friends before becoming visibly homeless.

Although the old stereotype of the public inebriate does not reflect the diversity of homelessness in the 1980s, alcohol abuse and alcoholism are still the most frequently diagnosed medical problems among homeless men (more than 40 percent). Substance abuse with drugs other than alcohol also appears to be more prevalent among homeless adults than among the general population, as is "comorbidity"—that is, multiple problems in the same individual such as alcoholism and mental illness.

The homeless have also been stereotyped as uniformly mentally ill, in part because *severe* disorders such as schizophrenia are conspicuously overrepresented among homeless individuals on the street. Most studies of mental illness among the homeless reveal that 30 to 40 percent of the adults show evidence of some type of major mental disorder; 15 to 25 percent acknowledge having been hospitalized for psychiatric care in the past. These rates are several times higher than those of the general population (Chapter 3).

Why Do People Become Homeless?

The answer to this seemingly simple question is quite complex. Among the many causes of homelessness, the committee identified three major, interrelated factors that, in the face of a relatively strong economy, have contributed to the increased number of homeless people in this decade:

1. *Housing*—The supply of housing units for people with low incomes has decreased considerably, while the number of people needing such housing has increased.
2. *Income and employment*—There has been a tightening of the eligibility criteria for public assistance programs (especially locally funded general relief), as well as a decline in the purchasing power of such benefits for those who do establish eligibility. This reduction in benefits comes at a time when the number of people living in poverty has increased.
3. *Deinstitutionalization*—The policy of deinstitutionalization, which characterizes the way state mental health systems have been administered since the early 1960s, is clearly a contributing factor; in addition, a policy of noninstitutionalization—that is, not admitting people for psychiatric care except for very brief periods of time—has further exacerbated the problems of mentally ill homeless adults. Both policies were based upon the assumption that treatment, rehabilitation, and appropriate residential placement would be provided in the community. This has not happened anywhere near the extent originally envisioned. Similar attitudes regarding extended confinement have come to characterize policy toward general hospitals and correctional, rehabilitation, and mental retardation facilities.

One result of these factors is that the system for providing temporary shelter for people who are homeless has been burdened beyond its capacity, despite enormous expansion in the last few years; people are staying in these emergency facilities for many months, not only a few days or weeks.

What Are the Health Problems of the Homeless?

Homeless people experience illnesses and injuries to a much greater extent than does the population as a whole. The committee identified three sets of health problems that specifically relate to homelessness:

1. Some health problems can cause a person to become homeless, for example, injury on the job resulting in the loss of employment and

income, severe mental illness, alcoholism, drug abuse, and, more recently, AIDS (acquired immune deficiency syndrome).

2. Other health problems result from homelessness, for example, problems resulting from exposure, such as hypothermia; problems resulting from not being able to lie down, such as vascular and skin disorders of the legs and feet; and problems resulting from specific hazards of the homeless life-style, such as trauma from being mugged or raped on the streets.

3. Many health problems require treatment that is made more complicated or impossible by the fact that the patient is homeless. Almost all illnesses and injuries fall within this category, and the difficulty encountered in attempting to treat even minor ailments when the patient is homeless is one of the major issues facing health care providers. One example would be the dietary limitations and the medication regimen that are part of the routine care of hypertension, a problem of particular significance among those past middle age and among blacks. Medication can rarely be taken as prescribed, and the sodium content of food derived from soup kitchens cannot be controlled. A simpler example would be the frequent order to "rest in bed"; this is virtually impossible if one does not have a bed, and very difficult at best if one must give up one's bed in a shelter every morning and wait until evening to be reassigned a bed.

What Other Problems Do Homeless People Have with Health Care?

The primary problem that homeless people have with health care is access, both financial and physical. With regard to financial access, homeless people generally face the same problems as do other poor and near-poor people: eligibility requirements for financial assistance, benefit levels well below the current market price for health care, and a reluctance of health care providers to supply low-cost treatment (especially in specialties like obstetrics, for which malpractice premiums are extremely high). Recent legislation has begun to eliminate one of the most serious obstacles to financial access for homeless people, that is, the requirement for a fixed address as a prerequisite for determining eligibility for public health care benefits. Depending on the state and the city, however, many homeless people—especially single, nondisabled adult individuals—are simply not eligible for such benefits.

With regard to physical access, those obstacles that often prevent the domiciled poor from obtaining health care prove to be still more difficult for the homeless. Hospitals, clinics, and mental health centers often are located far from the districts of cities where homeless people congregate.

The primary means of getting to health care programs is public transportation, which homeless people often cannot afford. In addition, if they do get to such programs, the long wait for services may mean that they miss the deadline when they must be back at the shelter to sign up for a bed for the night. Given a forced choice between treatment and a shelter for the night, shelter invariably becomes a first priority.

Responding to the health care needs of the homeless is more difficult than serving the medically indigent population generally. Personnel need special training and support for working with people who often are very distrustful, lack a network of social supports, and have a multiplicity of medical and social needs.

What Is Being Done About the Health Problems of Homeless People?

During the course of the study, members of the committee and the staff observed many commendable, well-utilized (and often overextended) health care and health care-related programs for homeless people throughout the country. Meetings were held with local officials, service providers, volunteers, and advocates for the homeless; numerous reports of other programs were evaluated. Of particular interest were the efforts of the 19 Robert Wood Johnson Foundation-Pew Memorial Trust Health Care for the Homeless projects, because they represented a particular targeted approach to providing health care services to homeless people. Moreover, while this study was in progress, Congress passed and the President signed into law the Stewart B. McKinney Homeless Assistance Act (P.L. 100-77), which provides new funding for a range of services, including general health and mental health care, in an effort to help the homeless (U.S. Congress, House, 1987).

However, even the most energetic health care worker is repeatedly confronted with the reality that poor and homeless people have trouble separating a specific need, such as health and mental health care, from the other activities needed for survival, such as securing housing and food. The committee concluded that even if the health care services that are clearly needed by so many of the homeless were widely available and accessible, the impact of such services would be severely restricted as long as the patients remained on the streets or in emergency shelters.

CONCLUSIONS AND RECOMMENDATIONS

Five Critical Observations

The fundamental problem encountered by homeless people—lack of a stable residence—has a direct and deleterious impact on health. Not only does homelessness cause health problems, it perpetuates and exacerbates poor health by seriously impeding efforts to treat disease and reduce disability.

Although the urgent need for focused health care and other prompt interventions is readily recognized, the committee found that the health problems of the homeless are inextricably intertwined with broad social and economic problems that require multifaceted, long-term approaches for their resolution. In spite of the limitations brought about by the committee's charge and the limitations of the committee's resources in its ability to formulate detailed recommendations to deal with the root causes of homelessness, the committee believes that those who seek solutions to the homelessness problem itself and to its attendant health-related problems must take into consideration the five critical observations described below.

1. More than anything else, homeless people need stable residences.

The health problems of homeless people that differ from those of other poor people are directly related to their homeless state. Homelessness is a risk factor that predisposes people to a variety of health problems and complicates treatment. The committee considers that decent housing is not only socially desirable but is necessary for the prevention of disease and the promotion of health. Yet the number of housing units for people with low incomes has been steadily decreasing since 1981, while the number of people needing such housing has been increasing during that same period.

2. People need income levels that make housing affordable, both to reduce and to prevent homelessness.

The issue of affordable housing has two sides: On one side is the supply of housing at a given price; on the other is the amount of money an individual or family has with which to pay rent. The committee observed that in many communities neither employment at the current minimum wage nor welfare benefits for those who are eligible provide enough income for them to acquire adequate housing. Given the irreducible economic cost of housing in those communities, income adequacy must also be addressed if homelessness and its attendant health problems are to be prevented or remedied.

3. Supportive services are necessary for some homeless people who require assistance in establishing and maintaining a stable residence.

Although the main issue is housing, for some homeless people, such as the chronically mentally ill, the mentally retarded, the physically disabled, those with histories of alcohol and drug abuse, the very young, and the very old, housing alone may not be sufficient. They need the kind of social support systems and appropriate health care that would allow them to maintain themselves in the community. Effective discharge planning, outreach services, and casework are necessary to identify needs and to ensure that these needs are met. With the proper support systems, many will outgrow their need for therapeutic milieus and specialized housing and will eventually become self-reliant. For some, however, the need may be lifelong.

4. Ensuring access to health care for the homeless should be part of a broad initiative to ensure access to health care for all those who are unable to pay.

In its deliberations, the committee examined ways to increase and to try to ensure access to health care for the homeless as a special group. It concluded, on both ethical and practical grounds, that a targeted approach was inappropriate in the long run. The committee found that, as a practical matter, those who provide health care services to homeless people also encounter other poor, uninsured people seeking access to health care. Moreover, as discussed in Chapter 2, the boundary between the homeless and the nonhomeless is thin and permeable. Although there are some chronically homeless people, many poor people slip in and out of homelessness. Extending health care services to the homeless while continuing to deny them to the domiciled poor is, thus, not only administratively impractical and bureaucratically cumbersome but also ethically difficult for those who provide or finance health care services. The committee agrees with the President's Commission for the Study of Ethical Problems in Medicine and Biomedical and Behavioral Research (1983) that the federal government has an obligation regarding access to needed health care:

> When equity occurs through the operation of private forces, there is no need for government involvement, but the ultimate responsibility for ensuring that society's obligation is met, through a combination of public and private sector arrangements, rests with the federal government.

5. Short-term solutions will not resolve what has clearly become a long-term problem.

The immediate and desperate need for shelter and food has overridden attempts to design and implement policies that might provide some long-term solutions. In the committee's view, what is needed now is planning and action at the federal, state, and local levels to coordinate and ensure the continuity of appropriate services and housing for homeless people. Although short-term, problem-specific approaches provide essential and sometimes lifesaving services, the committee does not believe that they will result in major enduring change.

Keeping these five observations in mind, the committee offers some recommendations about preventing and reducing homelessness before turning to recommendations focused on the immediate health care and other service needs of homeless people.

Preventing and Reducing Homelessness and Its Related Health Problems

As expressed throughout this report, health care and other services, including temporary shelters, can only help relieve some of the symptoms and consequences of homelessness. Coordinated efforts to address housing, income maintenance, and discharge planning are needed to prevent and reduce homelessness.

Housing

The problem of homelessness will persist and grow in the United States until the diminution and deterioration of housing units for people with low-incomes are reversed and affordable housing is made more widely available. Because of recent media attention to the refusal of certain homeless people to reside in institutional domiciles, there may be a misconception that homeless people will reject offers of decent and appropriate housing. There are no known studies that prove that if affordable housing were provided to homeless people they would use it, but several reports of the U.S. Conference of Mayors (1986a,b; 1987) regarding shelter utilization in excess of capacity support the belief that if such housing were available, the great majority of homeless people would surely accept it.

This is not a report on housing, nor was this committee made up of housing experts.* However, in light of the frequency with which the subject of housing arose during the course of this study, the committee makes the following observations:

1. For nearly five decades, beginning with the National Housing Act of 1938, the federal government has acknowledged, as a matter of explicit policy, its obligation to help ensure that every American family has access to decent housing. Because of the retreat from that commitment over the last several years, there has been a dramatic increase in the number of homeless people. The committee believes that if the health problems caused by homelessness are to be prevented, this commitment to housing should be reaffirmed.

2. Increasing the number of housing units for low-income people

---

* For a thoughtful analysis of this very complicated set of issues, see Alliance Housing Council (1988).

obviously requires major budgetary commitments. The lack of funds, however, is only one of several impediments to augmenting the housing supply. Among the nonfiscal issues that must be addressed are the impact of zoning regulations, real estate tax exemptions as incentives or disincentives to construct low-cost housing, local building construction standards, and the need for greater communication and coordination between the public agencies responsible for the disposition of abandoned housing and the public and private agencies that seek to help the homeless and ensure an adequate supply of affordable housing.

3. Many individuals and families only require a stable place to live, but some, especially the mentally ill, alcohol and drug abusers, the physically handicapped, and those with chronic and debilitating diseases, need housing and an array of professionally supervised supportive services in order to remain in the community—and, in many cases, to enable a transition to independent living. The committee believes that supportive housing programs for homeless people with disabilities are likely to be cost-effective and may lead to a reduction in future public expenditures; eventually, they may also enable these individuals to become economically productive citizens. Although there has long been a commitment to provide specialized housing (in the Community Mental Health Centers Act of 1962 [P.L. 88-164], for example, and implicitly in state governments' deinstitutionalization policies), the federal and state governments have not lived up to this commitment.

4. The Emergency Assistance program plays an important role in the provision of housing, especially as it relates to homeless families. In the committee's opinion, major aspects of this program that need to be reassessed include voluntary versus mandatory participation by the states, the use of Emergency Assistance funds to prevent—rather than simply to alleviate—homelessness, and the period of time and type of facilities (hotel rooms versus apartments) for which Emergency Assistance funds can be used. This reassessment is especially urgent in light of the present high prevalence of homelessness and the widespread expectation that the problem will get worse before it gets better.

Income and Benefits

Throughout its deliberations, the committee was impressed by the fact that improvements in income maintenance and other benefit programs for people in poverty would help appreciably in preventing and reducing homelessness and its related health problems. In this section the committee offers some observations and conclusions, urges the implementation of existing legislation, and recommends that some new legislation be considered.

The committee observes that a growing number of people with full-time jobs are becoming homeless. During its site visits around the country, the committee heard numerous references to people who are working but who cannot afford the most basic form of housing, not even a single room (see Chapters 1 and 2). This suggests that the relation of the minimum wage level to housing costs should be reexamined.

The committee also observed that many homeless people do not qualify for federally supported entitlement programs such as Medicaid and food stamps. Moreover, for those who do qualify, the benefit levels are so low as to make it impossible for them to obtain adequate housing or services. The committee did not find that there is any substantial justification for major geographic variations in eligibility standards. There may be a basis for some differences in benefit levels because of regional variations in the cost of living, but the dramatic differences in benefit levels from state to state identified in Chapter 4 do not appear to be justified.

Therefore, we recommend **that the federal government should review all federally funded entitlement programs in order to create rational eligibility standards and establish benefit levels based upon the actual cost of living in a specific region.** The committee commends state courts, such as those in Massachusetts and New York, for their recent decisions holding that entitlement benefits should be great enough to enable the recipients to afford that for which the benefits are intended, whether it be housing, food, or health care (see Chapter 5), and recommends that this approach be adopted by other states and the federal government in establishing benefit levels.

In terms of eligibility for benefits, the committee found that the 1986 federal legislation requiring the development of procedures to ensure that the absence of a permanent address does not constitute a barrier to receipt of cash assistance, food stamps, Medicaid, and other benefits has yet to be fully implemented. **The committee urges prompt, uniform implementation of these procedures. Furthermore, the committee recommends that state and local governments reexamine their documentation requirements for public benefit programs** to ensure that they, too, do not impose unrealistic requirements on homeless people (Chapter 2).

The committee observed that some homeless people who are eligible for income and other benefits are unaware of their eligibility or are unable to secure them. Augmented outreach efforts to identify and assist the homeless and those at risk of becoming homeless (especially those about to be discharged from institutions) could reduce and prevent homelessness (see the section Health Care and Related Services in this chapter for a more complete discussion of outreach). The committee recommends the following:

• The effects of extending the presumptive eligibility guidelines for Supplemental Security Income (SSI) to include disabled homeless people (especially homeless people who have been discharged from a mental hospital within the preceding 90 days [Chapters 2 and 4]) should be evaluated in order to assess the costs and impact on the rates of homelessness.

• The effects of the current federal regulation that mandates a 33.3 percent cash reduction in benefits for SSI recipients who live with other people should be carefully assessed. Questions such as the following need to be addressed: To what extent is the regulation contributing to homelessness by deterring people from sharing housing? Given the high cost of even the most basic forms of shelter services, would there be savings that would result from removing this regulation and, if so, what would the magnitude of the savings be?

Finally, the committee recommends that **serious consideration** be given to the following two changes in the Medicaid system:

• **Medicaid eligibility should be decoupled from eligibility for other benefits, and a national minimum eligibility standard should be established for Medicaid** (Chapter 4). These changes would enhance access to health care for certain vulnerable groups—such as families whose Medicaid eligibility is lost if they lose Aid to Families with Dependent Children (AFDC) benefits.

• **Medicaid regulations should be amended to provide reimbursement for community-based services (e.g., day treatment and case management) for homeless people with psychiatric or physical disabilities in order to assist them in community integration (Chapters 1, 3, and 4) and reduce current incentives for institutionalization.**

Discharge Planning

Inadequate discharge planning coupled with inadequate community-based support and housing can cause homelessness. State, local, and private mental hospitals; inpatient substance abuse facilities; facilities for mentally retarded and developmentally disabled people; general hospitals; nursing homes; and correctional facilities all share a common responsibility to help arrange access for their clients or patients to appropriate and affordable postinstitutional living arrangements, including supportive services when necessary. Three sets of variables appear to affect the likelihood of postinstitutional placement most frequently:

1. Whether a person was homeless at the time of admission or became homeless during his or her institutional stay.
2. Whether there is a supply of affordable housing and supportive services or whether such housing or services are virtually nonexistent.

3. Whether even a basic minimum effort to locate housing and services is expended by the institution or whether that task is inappropriately delegated to shelters.

Some people become homeless because the institutions that are responsible for their care fail to ensure that they can maintain themselves in the community after they are discharged. Although the committee recognizes that there is a shortage of affordable housing, it believes that more effective discharge planning will help homeless people have greater access to that which is available. (On the related issue of the need for additional services for those who require posthospital nursing care, see the section Convalescent Services later in this chapter.) Just as it is inappropriate for a person who is not sick to remain in a hospital, so is it inappropriate for institutions simply to discharge people to shelters or to the streets without having made even the most basic efforts to find alternative living arrangements.

The committee recommends that public and private institutions adopt and observe discharge planning processes that ensure in advance of discharge—to the extent possible—that clients have suitable living arrangements and necessary supportive services. To help increase the availability of adequate postdischarge arrangements, such institutions must work to improve communications and coordination with organizations that provide postdischarge ambulatory care, home health care services, and other relevant community agencies and organizations (Chapter 5).

Moreover, **federal and state agencies that provide financing to hospitals and other relevant institutions should extend to all beneficiaries of public programs the standards for discharge planning that now apply to Medicare patients.**

Health Care and Related Services

The committee found that the most effective health care and other services for homeless people are those that recognize the special needs and characteristics of the homeless. With this in mind, the committee recommends that the following general strategies be adopted:

• **services should be provided on a voluntary basis**, respectful of individual privacy and dignity;
• **intensive efforts should be made to engage homeless people by reaching out to them at the places where they congregate;** this requires appropriately skilled and trained health care professionals who can link clients to and provide continuity of services in community-based health care centers, free-standing clinics, hospital outpatient departments, and other existing providers of services;

- health care providers should be trained in the special problems of patient engagement and communication;
- health care providers should be trained in the diagnosis, treatment, and follow-up of those conditions that are especially prevalent among homeless people;
- techniques should be developed to address the particular difficulties homeless people have in maintaining medication or dietary regimens; and
- ways should be developed for homeless patients to obtain needed medicines, medical supplies, or equipment.

In many respects, homeless people have the same health care needs as other poor people. A high prevalence of acute and chronic diseases is found among the homeless, so health care needs to be available and accessible. **The committee recommends that serious efforts be made to identify those in need of treatment and to encourage intervention at the earliest appropriate time in order to avoid unnecessary deterioration in their health status. Such health care should include, for example, either by direct provision or by contractual agreement, primary health care services such as pediatric care (including well-baby care and immunizations), prenatal care, dental care, testing and treatment for sexually transmitted diseases, birth control, screening and treatment for hypertension, podiatric care, and mental health services.**

Outreach

As discussed throughout this report, homeless people have multiple service needs. The provision of such services is complicated by the state of being homeless. Although there have been occasional reports of homeless people refusing services, data from the 19 Johnson-Pew projects indicate that, when properly approached, the homeless welcome services. In fact, demand for services has exceeded earlier projections for the utilization of both health care services and shelter space (U.S. Conference of Mayors, 1986a; Wright and Weber, 1987).

Aggressive outreach efforts and coordinated case management are crucial to successful service provision to homeless people. Intensive efforts to identify homeless people who are in need of health care and other services, to determine eligibility for benefits, to encourage acceptance of appropriate treatment, and to facilitate receipt of services are needed.

The committee recommends that the Social Security Administration substantially expand its outreach efforts, already mandated by statute, to include sites at which homeless people congregate. Special efforts should be made to expedite the assessment of eligibility for disability benefits of chronically mentally ill people about to be discharged from institutions. For example, consideration should be given to:

- developing descriptive materials on the current prerelease program for use by the Social Security Administration's (SSA) local offices;
- requiring a specific period within which state agencies must file and act upon disability applications received as part of the prerelease program;
- amending SSI regulations to permit applications for SSI to be completed and processed (either granted or denied) before a person's discharge;
- requiring local SSA personnel to routinely seek, accept, and process disability applications from patients in state mental hospitals; SSA workers should be trained to become effective liaisons with institutions in their area; and
- establishing a system for collecting national, regional, and local data on approval or denial of SSI disability claims of individuals in institutions.

Given the apparent effectiveness of the Veterans Administration's (VA) pilot project to reach homeless veterans suffering from mental illness, the committee recommends the following:

- **Additional funding should be appropriated to allow the expansion of the outreach program to those facilities that did not receive outreach staff under the original pilot project and, when necessary, to allow additional staffing for those facilities serving geographic areas with a high prevalence of homeless people. Furthermore, ways should be found to expand the VA's outreach effort to include homeless veterans who are not chronically mentally ill.**
- Because the VA has already shown itself to be willing to assist in preventing homelessness by serving those "at serious risk" of becoming homeless, **the VA should consider expanding its efforts to include outreach to such institutional settings as mental hospitals, acute-care hospitals, and prisons so that assessment and placement can be arranged before people are released from such facilities.**
- The VA has given recognition to the possibility that some homeless veterans are "wary about coming to a hospital" (Rosenheck et al., 1987). **It is recommended that the VA consider alternatives to having psychiatric and medical assessments done at a medical facility and to determine whether changes will increase the number of veterans for whom follow-up care and placement is actually accomplished.**
- **The VA should increase its efforts to publicize its outreach program to providers of non-health care-related services to the homeless; as the outreach program becomes more fully established, the VA should pursue more formal means of linkage with other providers of services.**

• During several of its site visits, including a site visit to the community placement program at the VA Medical Center in Lexington, Kentucky, committee members heard frequent reference to a lack of appropriate supportive residential programs for veterans from the Vietnam era. Programs such as the community placement program, although rendering excellent service to the older veterans from World War II and the Korean conflict, were not seen as appropriate for the younger, more active Vietnam veterans. Because the initial outreach effort has determined that a majority of the homeless veterans whom they have seen were from the Vietnam era, **the VA should place a greater priority on developing programs that are more appropriate for meeting the needs of younger veterans.**

Casework

After food and shelter, effective social casework is the fundamental service needed for nearly every homeless person. Such an approach, under appropriate professional supervision, is essential because of the multiple problems homeless people encounter in the complex interactions among employment, personal behavior, and public and private benefit and service programs. A coordinated local effort that enables public and private agencies to improve their communications would increase the likelihood that homeless people would use the programs and services to which they are entitled. In many communities, the creation of such a network will take time. Therefore, in the interim, the committee recommends the following:

• **Ways should be found for providers of services to the homeless, including, for example, shelters, soup kitchens, and drop-in centers, to make casework services available to all clients willing to accept them.** Such intensive case management should focus on enrollment for benefits, services management, health care management, services coordination, and vocational assistance. These efforts should be aimed at ending the client's homelessness and facilitating his or her reintegration into the community.

• **Casework services must be adequately funded.** Federal, state, local, and voluntary agencies that fund services to the homeless should be encouraged to provide adequate resources. For example:

1. For AFDC families, Federal Financial Participation for the administrative costs of casework should be increased as an incentive to states to increase their support (Chapter 4).
2. The Protection and Advocacy for Mentally Ill Individuals Act (P.L. 99-319), which currently applies only to mentally ill people in residential settings, should be amended to support protection and advocacy

services for homeless people who are mentally ill, irrespective of their location.

Nutrition

Nutrition is of particular concern to the health and well-being of the homeless, who are usually too poor to purchase adequate food and who have no place to prepare it. For those who receive food in soup kitchens and shelters, they get what is available without regard for special dietary needs. Homeless infants, children, and chronically ill adults are especially vulnerable to nutritional problems. Therefore, the committee recommends the following:

• **Providers of food to the homeless, such as operators of shelters, soup kitchens, and food pantries, should be educated in and encouraged to follow principles of sound nutrition and the special nutritional needs of the homeless** (Chapter 3).

• **The recently established practice of permitting food stamps to be used at soup kitchens and other feeding sites should be extended to permit the use of food stamps to purchase prepared foods from restaurants and elsewhere** (Chapters 1, 2, and 4).

• **Because even the most prudent and imaginative parents in homeless families cannot provide adequate nutrition for young children at existing levels of food stamp benefits, such benefits should be recalculated to reflect realistic expenses to meet nutritional requirements.**

• The Special Supplemental Food Program for Women, Infants, and Children (WIC) provides food assistance and nutritional screening to women and children below 185 percent of the poverty level; however, funding for this program is not adequate to provide such benefits to all those who are eligible (U.S. Congress, House, Committee on Ways and Means, 1987). Because many homeless women are pregnant and a growing number of homeless people are children, it is especially important that **the WIC Program be strengthened in order to address comprehensively the nutritional needs of pregnant women and young children.**

Mental Health, Alcoholism, and Drug Abuse

Alcohol-related problems and mental disorders are the two most prevalent health problems among homeless adult individuals, and drug abuse appears to be on the increase. Since the early 1980s the National Institute of Mental Health, the National Institute on Alcohol Abuse and Alcoholism, and the National Institute on Drug Abuse have each funded programmatic and basic research in these areas as they relate to homelessness. More recent programs, such as the community mental health services demonstration projects for homeless individuals who are chronically mentally ill and the community demonstration projects for the treatment of homeless individuals who abuse alcohol and drugs (as mandated by Sections 612 and 613 of the Stewart B. McKinney Homeless Assistance Act), have significant potential for combating the major problems of these populations. Increased efforts to aid other homeless people, whether they are individuals or families, should not be at the expense of these existing programs.

In recent years, the trend has been to separate programs that serve the mentally ill, alcoholics, and drug abusers. However, because there is growing evidence of dual and multiple diagnoses among these populations (see Chapters 1 and 3) and because there are certain basic similarities in efforts to provide treatment, those recommendations that address elements common to programs that treat individuals with all three diagnoses are identified before those recommendations relating to individuals with a specific diagnosis. In seeking to resolve the very complicated interrelationships among homelessness and mental illness, alcoholism, and drug abuse, the following services should be included:

• **targeted outreach services** directed at homeless individuals suffering from mental illness, alcoholism, or drug abuse;

• **supportive living environments** encompassing programs ranging from the most structured to the least structured; this is necessary so that as the individual improves, progress can be made through several stages of decreasing support and on to independent living, when possible (some will need various support services throughout their lifetimes);

• **treatment and rehabilitation services** appropriate to the individual's diagnosis and functional level; this must be a range of such services so that, again, the individual who improves can become less dependent on such programs while moving to self-sufficiency; and

• **specialized case management** provided by professionals who not only understand the complexities of these illnesses as they relate to homelessness but who also understand the complexities of systems that seek to provide mental health, alcoholism, and drug abuse services.

In addressing the issues of the mentally ill, alcoholic, or drug-abusing homeless, the committee saw repeated reference in the literature and heard from those actively engaged with these populations that **greater communication, consultation, and continuing liaison** between providers of services are needed. This is especially true for homeless adult individuals who suffer from more than one of these diagnoses, who suffer from one such diagnosis along with some other disabling condition (e.g., a physical disability), or who suffer from one form of substance abuse while using other substances as "enhancers." It is critical that **people suffering from**

dual or multiple diagnoses (physical illnesses, mental disorders, and addictions) not be left unserved or underserved because of the overspecialization of treatment programs. It is far more cost-effective to coordinate existing services than it would be to create new treatment programs directed at each possible combination of diagnoses.

With regard to specific problem areas, the committee offers the following conclusions and recommendations.

Mental health. The institutional mental health system appears to be an inappropriate place to focus policymakers' attention in trying to resolve the broad problems of homelessness. Proposals purporting to resolve the problem of homelessness by changing commitment laws or by substantially relaxing standards for admission to mental hospitals are misguided and lead to an erroneous belief that the mental health system alone can correct a problem for which all systems bear a responsibility. The central issue in mental health care is the lack of an adequate supply of appropriate and high-quality services throughout the mental health care system, including state psychiatric centers and psychiatric units in acute-care hospitals and in the community. **The committee recommends that the first priority in addressing the problems of the mentally ill homeless must be to ensure the adequate availability of clinical services (including professionally supervised supportive housing arrangements) at all levels.** Of these, the most serious deficiency between supply and demand—and that which is most directly linked to homelessness—is at the community level.

Alcoholism and alcohol abuse. In addition to an inadequate supply of those services cited earlier (outreach, supportive living, treatment, and case management) as they relate to homeless individuals suffering from alcoholism, the committee notes a serious shortage of services directed toward the specific relationship between alcoholism and homelessness. In light of the fact that studies have shown that homeless alcoholics are at significantly greater risk of certain health problems (e.g, tuberculosis and hypothermia) than nonalcoholic homeless individuals and that alcoholism may become an integral part of the life-style of homelessness, the treatment of alcoholism among the homeless in the same manner and at the same locations as those for the domiciled alcoholic may not be the most effective. **The committee recommends that both public and private agencies and organizations treating alcoholism develop programs specifically for the homeless and those alcoholics at high risk of becoming homeless.** The committee notes that recent developments such as alcohol-free living environments (e.g., "sober hotels") and programs that combine both medical and social approaches to the treatment of alcoholism appear to be especially promising.

Drug abuse.   While not yet as prevalent as mental illness or alcoholism among the homeless single adult population, drug abuse, especially among younger adult men, is increasing. In particular, because of its close correlation with AIDS, the issue of intravenous drug abuse has come to greater public awareness, as has the inability of the existing drug abuse treatment system to respond to the increased demand for treatment services. **The committee joins with others in recommending that treatment services for intravenous drug abusers be increased to the extent that anyone desiring such services can be accommodated.** The cost of such services is relatively minor when compared with the costs of treatment and care for those physical diseases associated with intravenous drug abuse, such as AIDS and hepatitis.

The prevalence rates for mental illness, alcoholism, and drug abuse are much lower among adults who are members of homeless families than among homeless adults who are not, but the fact remains that such health problems are more prevalent among homeless parents than among the general population. Furthermore, the long-term impact on treatment programs and social service systems resulting from the effect of the parents' problems on the children could become very costly in the future. Both in terms of their value as a preventive measure and as the more cost-effective approach to contain the need for such services years from now, the committee recommends that **the relevant federal, state, and local agencies, as well as the relevant private not-for-profit agencies, should begin to examine alternate ways to treat mental illness, alcoholism, and drug abuse among homeless parents, giving due consideration to the limitations of time and mobility inherent in a parent's role.** In addition, **Congress should consider extending the provisions of the Stewart B. McKinney Homeless Assistance Act of 1987 that currently deal with mental illness and the treatment of alcoholism and drug abuse in individual adults to cover homeless parents, children, and adolescents as well.**

Convalescent Services

The committee recommends that Federal Emergency Management Administration funds and other funds be made available, in every community, to support the development and operation of facilities in which homeless people can safely convalesce from subacute illnesses or transient exacerbations of chronic illnesses, or to which they can safely and appropriately be discharged from acute-care facilities. As described in Chapter 3, adequate health care for homeless people is often made impossible by the simple absence of a secure place for them to convalesce. There is a clear need for facilities that provide appropriate rest and nutrition as well as limited personal care for periods generally not in excess of 30 days.

Other Services

The Stewart B. McKinney Homeless Assistance Act of 1987 (P.L. 100-77) creates a federal Interagency Council on the Homeless and charges it to "review all federal activities and programs to assist homeless individuals." This study committee, in the course of its many site visits, observed several programs that are partially federally funded. For example, the Cardinal Medeiros Center in Boston receives some of its funding under the Older Americans Act (P.L. 89-73), and the Larkin Street Youth Center in San Francisco receives some of its support under the Runaway and Homeless Youth Act (P.L. 98-473). Often, these programs are not targeted directly toward, or identified with, the homeless. In some cases, such funding is due to expire along with the enabling legislation.

The committee recommends that the interagency council mandated by P.L. 100-77 give high priority to its review of all programs that might be of assistance in helping subpopulations among the homeless, irrespective of whether such programs are specifically directed toward helping homeless people. The council should:

- conduct an extensive review of such support programs, primarily to identify programs that are providing or that could provide help to subpopulations among the homeless;
- review joint federal–state efforts, such as state veterans homes with partial federal funding, that, although not targeted directly to the homeless, might help many homeless people;
- publicize successful efforts to help the homeless as a means of encouraging other groups to develop similar programs in their communities; and
- consider ways and means of extending or enhancing the funding for programs that are deemed effective in relieving or preventing homelessness until the current prevalence of homelessness is substantially reduced.

Special Needs of Homeless Children and Their Parents

The committee feels strongly that the growing phenomenon of homeless children is nothing short of a national disgrace that must be treated with the urgency that such a situation demands. The committee has chosen to offer a number of recommendations relating to services for homeless children, only because it believes that the fundamental reforms to income maintenance programs, the child welfare system, and foster care programs will take a number of years to implement and that, in the interim, the tens of thousands of homeless children are in urgent need of a broad range of services.

Recent studies have documented that the majority of homeless children of various ages manifest delayed development, serious symptoms of depression and anxiety, or learning problems (Bassuk and Rubin, 1987; Bassuk and Rosenberg, 1988). These are early signs that vulnerability is turning into disability for these youngsters; efforts by human service professionals may be able to reverse these liabilities and to prevent further damage. There is now a considerable body of evidence demonstrating the benefits to disadvantaged and disorganized families of intensive family-oriented services; such approaches are characterized by flexibility in meeting families' multiple needs and by specific aids such as developmental day care, infant stimulation programs, parental counseling, and Head Start. Such intensive intervention efforts—even if expensive to begin with—have proved to be cost-effective in the long run (Schorr, 1988). Because the homeless are an especially vulnerable subpopulation of poor people, the committee believes that such programs would be of similar benefit to this group. It recognizes that because the population of homeless families includes some of the most hopeless and alienated among the poor—and because they are more likely to move from place to place—there may be obstacles to participation in such programs; therefore, the committee recommends the following:

• **Federal support for enriched day care and Head Start programs should be expanded and coupled with the development of outreach efforts to encourage homeless parents to take advantage of enrichment programs for themselves, their infants, and their young children.**

• **Local and state agencies that receive federal Head Start funds should be mandated to develop plans to identify and evaluate homeless children of preschool age and to provide them with appropriate services.**

• **Federal support for local and state education agencies should be conditional on the adoption of plans for identifying, evaluating, and serving homeless children of school age, including needed transportation services. These plans should include specific mechanisms for liaison and service coordination among educational, shelter, and social service agencies** (Chapters 1 and 3).

• **Apart from any mandates that may accompany federal support, community agencies—acting in concert with school boards, local philanthropies, and other organizations—should be encouraged to develop programs of family-oriented services for homeless children and their parents. Such services need to be both intensive and comprehensive.**

Shelters

In the committee's view, **shelters should not become a permanent network of new institutions or substandard human service organizations.**

As desirable housing is developed, the shelter system should be substantially reduced in size and returned to its original intent to provide short-term crisis intervention. In the interim, the committee recommends that action be taken to reduce the hazards to the health of homeless people that may be created or exacerbated by shelters.

- **The federal government should convene a panel of appropriate experts to develop model standards for life and fire safety, sanitation, and disease prevention in shelters and other facilities in which 10 or more homeless people are domiciled.** This code should be predicated on the recognition that shelters, welfare hotels, and the like should provide short-term, emergency housing and are not satisfactory longer term substitutes for housing and other services (Chapters 2 and 3).

- Once a model code is developed and after a reasonable amount of time has passed for compliance to be obtained, **the federal government should adopt the standards as a condition for receipt of Emergency Assistance payments or other federal assistance, including Federal Emergency Management Agency funds.** However, Federal Emergency Management Agency funds should be made available to assist existing shelters to achieve compliance with the standards.

- **The federal government should disseminate the model code to encourage voluntary compliance.** State and local governments should be encouraged to adopt it on a mandatory basis for shelters that do not receive federal funds but that do receive funds from state and local governments.

- **Adequate provision must be made to shelter families as a unit.** The consequences of homelessness are serious enough without being worsened by family disruption.

- **In light of the increasing prevalence of sexually transmitted diseases, including AIDS, and unplanned pregnancies among the homeless, the committee recommends that shelters, particularly those used by younger single men, women, and adolescents, provide birth control counseling and services, including free condoms, to reduce the risks of these conditions** (Chapters 1 and 3). It is recognized that data on the effectiveness of these recommendations in shelter populations do not exist and that many individuals, including some providers of services, may have ethical or philosophical objections, but it is the consensus of the committee that this recommendation represents sound public health practice.

Volunteer Efforts

The provision of services to homeless people depends heavily on the efforts of volunteers. Even with the recommended expansion of federal, state, and local government support, volunteers will be needed. The committee believes that the extraordinary contributions of services to homeless people by volunteer professionals and laymen must be better recognized, encouraged, and rewarded. **Federal, state, and local governments and local United Way and other charitable agencies should work with service-providing organizations to improve their capacity to recruit, train, use, and recognize volunteers.** Universities should play a major role in providing support by using programs for the homeless as part of their training curricula, especially in social work, law, medicine, dentistry, nursing, optometry, and the allied health professions. Not only would this improve the quantity and quality of volunteer efforts, but it would also provide students with extraordinary learning experiences and make them more sympathetic to those whom they will serve during their careers. Hospitals and other health care facilities should be encouraged to provide in-kind support (including clinic space and medications) for volunteers in their communities who help the homeless. Health professionals and lawyers should be encouraged to provide *pro bono* services, and professional organizations on the national, state, and local levels should establish formal programs in support of such efforts and provide recognition of those who provide such services.

State insurance commissioners should take measures to prevent carriers of medical, professional, or institutional liability insurance from charging additional, excessive, or discriminatory premiums or refusing to provide coverage for health care providers who serve the homeless without adequate documented actuarial experience to justify such action. This is especially critical in regard to malpractice and liability insurance because it is already difficult to recruit volunteers and to create university affiliations for training in the settings in which homeless people are served; these programs can ill afford to bear the additional burden of excessive insurance premiums or the potential loss of coverage.

Research

Many questions about the health of the homeless remain unanswered. Research is needed to elucidate the health and mental health disorders of the homeless, the methods of providing health care, and the factors that affect accessibility.

The Johnson-Pew Health Care for the Homeless projects provide the only extensive data base on the general health condition of homeless people (Wright and Weber, 1987). The shortcomings of these data are that they document health problems in individuals seeking help at clinics and are based on presenting complaints rather than systematic health evaluations; therefore, hidden health problems are not included.

There are no longitudinal data that document the fate of homeless people. For example, it is a frequent observation that there are relatively few homeless people over the age of 50, but the reasons for this are unknown. Though there have been calls from many quarters for additional resources to meet the needs of homeless people, there is still a paucity of information as to the ways in which resources should be allocated.

Various subgroups of the homeless have different health service needs; to consider the homeless as a homogeneous population is to be mistaken. Research is needed to identify the various subgroups of homeless people and their particular problems and health service requirements. Regional variations are also important; the problems of displaced workers in rural areas or small towns of the South or Midwest can be very different from those of displaced factory workers in the eastern industrial cities, which have more diversified economies.

Specific disorders deserve particular attention by researchers in epidemiology and health care services. These include tuberculosis and AIDS. Alcoholism has traditionally been and continues to be the most prevalent single medical condition of homeless people; improved methods of outreach, detoxification, rehabilitation, and long-term maintenance should be developed and evaluated. Abuse of other drugs also needs further research. The National Institute of Mental Health and the Robert Wood Johnson Foundation are to be especially commended for the initiatives that they have taken in encouraging and supporting research in the financing, organization, and delivery of services to the severely mentally ill.

Public and private research funding organizations should encourage research into the dynamics of homelessness, the health problems of homeless people, and effective service provision strategies. Specifically, the following research is most critically needed:

- longitudinal studies of the natural history of homelessness;
- studies of the prevalence of acute and chronic diseases in homeless populations;
- the role of illness as a precipitant of homelessness and the ability of health care and social service systems to prevent this outcome;
- studies of the homeless population and the prevalence of infectious diseases (e.g., tuberculosis, hepatitis, and AIDS) and chronic disorders or disabilities (e.g., mental retardation and epilepsy);
- studies of effective treatment programs for homeless alcoholics;
- development and evaluation of programs for homeless people who are mentally ill; and
- studies of the effects of homelessness on the health and development of children and evaluation of strategies to prevent homelessness in families and to give additional support to homeless families.

REFERENCES

Alliance Housing Council. 1988. Housing and Homelessness. Washington, D.C.: National Alliance to End Homelessness.

Bassuk, E. L., and L. Rosenberg. 1988. Why does family homelessness occur? A case-control study. American Journal of Public Health 78(7):783–788.

Bassuk, E. L., and L. Rubin. 1987. Homeless children: A neglected population. American Journal of Orthopsychiatry 5(2):1–9.

President's Commission for the Study of Ethical Problems in Medicine and Biomedical and Behavioral Research. 1983. Securing Access to Health Care: The Ethical Implications of Differences in the Availability of Health Services, Volume 1. Washington, D.C.: U.S. Government Printing Office.

Rosenheck, R., P. Gallup, C. Leda, P. Leaf, R. Milstein, I. Voynick, P. Errera, L. Lehman, G. Koerber, and R. Murphy. 1987. Progress Report on the Veterans Administration Program for Homeless Chronically Mentally Ill Veterans. Washington, D.C.: Veterans Administration.

Schorr, L. B. 1988. Within Our Reach: Breaking the Cycle of Disadvantage. New York: Doubleday.

U.S. Conference of Mayors. 1986a. The Growth of Hunger, Homelessness, and Poverty in America's Cities in 1985: A 25-City Survey. Washington, D.C.: U.S. Conference of Mayors.

U.S. Conference of Mayors. 1986b. The Continued Growth of Hunger, Homelessness, and Poverty in America's Cities: 1986. A 25-City Survey. Washington, D.C.: U.S. Conference of Mayors.

U.S. Conference of Mayors. 1987. Status Report on Homeless Families in America's Cities: A 29-City Survey. Washington, D.C.: U.S. Conference of Mayors.

U.S. Congress, House. 1987. Stewart B. McKinney Homeless Assistance Act, Conference Report to accompany H.R. 558. Report 100-174. 100th Cong., 1st sess.

U.S. Congress, House, Committee on Ways and Means. 1987. Background material and data on programs within the jurisdiction of the Committee on Ways and Means. 100th Cong., 1st sess. March 6, 1987.

Wright, J. D., and E. Weber. 1987. Homelessness and Health. New York: McGraw-Hill.

APPENDIXES

A Legislative Efforts to Aid the Homeless

In 1983, Congress appropriated $100 million for emergency food and shelter to be funneled to community groups through the Federal Emergency Management Agency (FEMA). Since then it has appropriated $320 million more for this purpose and has made changes in federal housing assistance, food stamps, Medicaid, mental health, Aid to Families with Dependent Children (AFDC), Supplemental Security Income (SSI), veterans, job training, and other programs primarily to make them more accessible to the homeless. A brief summary of measures enacted since 1983 follows.

P.L. 98-8: With passage of the Emergency Jobs Appropriations Act of 1983, Congress appropriated $100 million for emergency food and shelter to be channeled to community-based groups through FEMA. Half of the funds were disseminated by a national board of volunteer organizations and the other half were allocated to the states as formula grants. The act also provided $125 million to the U.S. Department of Agriculture to purchase ($75 million) and distribute ($50 million) surplus food commodities to the needy. The new program was named the Temporary Emergency Food Assistance Program (TEFAP).

P.L. 98-94: The 1984 Department of Defense Authorization Act permitted military installations to make facilities available for shelters.

P.L.'s 98-151, 98-181, and 98-396: Various appropriations measures passed in 1984 gave FEMA an additional $110 million to be allocated for emergency food and shelter. P.L. 98-181 also provided $60 million for an emergency shelter program to be administered by the U.S. Department of Housing and Urban Development (HUD); however, these funds were

165

never expended. HUD testifies that Community Development Block Grant money was being used for the same purpose.

P.L. 98-288: The Domestic Volunteer Service Act Amendments of 1983 authorized the use of Volunteers in Service to America (VISTA) in projects to aid the homeless.

P.L.'s 99-88 and 99-160: Two appropriations acts passed in 1985 gave FEMA an additional $90 million to be allocated for emergency food and shelter.

P.L. 99-129: The Health Professions Training Assistance Act of 1985 directed the secretary of the U.S. Department of Health and Human Services (HHS) to arrange with the National Academy of Sciences for an Institute of Medicine study of the delivery of inpatient and outpatient health care services to homeless people.

P.L. 99-167: The 1986 Military Construction Authorization Act permitted military installations to make surplus bedding available to shelter operators.

P.L. 99-198: The Food Security Act of 1985 required state welfare offices to develop ways to issue food stamps to people with no permanent address. It also reauthorized TEFAP through fiscal year 1987 (FY87) again providing $50 million per year for distribution costs but imposing a cost-sharing requirement on distribution activities run at the state government level.

P.L. 99-570: As part of the Anti-Drug Abuse Act of 1986, Congress enacted the Homeless Eligibility Clarification Act that (1) removed the bar to food stamp eligibility for shelter residents and permitted the homeless to use food stamps to buy prepared meals from soup kitchens and shelters; (2) required the federal agencies responsible for Medicaid, AFDC, and SSI to develop methods to assess eligibility for, and make aid available to, people who do not have fixed home or mailing addresses; (3) prohibited the denial of veterans' benefits because of the lack of a mailing address; (4) required the Social Security Administration (SSA) to make regular visits to facilities for the homeless to take SSI and food stamp applications, and required SSA and the U.S Department of Agriculture to develop procedures to take SSI and food stamp applications from people about to be discharged from medical, penal, and other institutions; and (5) explicitly made the homeless eligible for state and local job training programs authorized by the Job Training Partnership Act and required that their job training be coordinated with education, training, and assistance available under other public programs.

The Veterans Administration and the U.S. Department of Agriculture have promulgated and adopted the mandated regulatory frameworks. They are effective retroactively to October 1986. SSA has issued revisions to its program operating manual; the Health Care Financing Administration published a new policy statement in February 1987 that implemented the provisions of P.L. 99-570.

P.L. 99-591:   As part of a continuing appropriations measure, $15 million was given to HUD to allocate in FY87 (under the title of the Homeless Housing Act of 1986) for housing demonstration projects affecting the homeless. The measure also gave FEMA an additional $70 million to be allocated for emergency food and shelter.

P.L. 99-660:   As part of an omnibus health care bill, Congress gave the National Institute of Mental Health (NIMH) specific authority to award grants for demonstration projects affecting the homeless mentally ill.

P.L. 100-6:   Congress passed a measure reallocating $50 million in disaster relief funds to programs aiding the homeless. So that these funds would be of some relief during the winter months, Congress passed H.J. Res. 102, a supplemental appropriations act permitting $45 million of the previously reallocated funds to be used for FEMA's emergency food and shelter program and the other $5 million to be used by the Veterans Administration (VA) to provide services to homeless mentally ill veterans. The administration initially opposed the transfer, arguing that it might jeopardize the disaster relief program and that the money would not reach the homeless in time to meet winter needs. The resolution also included language rejecting the administration's proposed deferral of $28.6 million for distribution costs under the U.S. Department of Agriculture's surplus food distribution program (TEFAP). Although considerable controversy emerged over the resolution after the Senate added language rejecting an imminent congressional pay raise, the resolution passed both houses of Congress and was signed into law on February 12, 1987.

P.L. 100-77:   The major homeless aid bill of the 100th Congress, H.R. 558, the Stewart B. McKinney Homeless Assistance Act of 1987, was signed into law on July 23, 1987. In a parallel action taken by Congress, a supplemental appropriations bill authorizing most of the funds for P.L. 100-77 was passed and signed into law on July 11, 1987.

The following are some highlights of this particular piece of legislation.

• Authorization of $200,000 for FY87 and $2.5 million to establish a 3-year Interagency Council on the Homeless, composed of most cabinet secretaries and the heads of several independent agencies.

• Authorization of $15 million for FY87 (in addition to funds already appropriated) and $124 million for FY88 for FEMA's emergency food and shelter program, which had been operating by way of appropriation language for the previous 4 years.

• Authorizations, with regard to HUD, for (1) $100 million in FY87 and $120 million in FY88 for state grants for emergency shelter and $80 million in FY87 and $100 million in FY88 for a supportive housing demonstration program (of which at least $20 million would be earmarked for projects that serve homeless families with children and at least $15 million for projects providing permanent housing for handicapped homeless people); the amounts that would be authorized for FY87 for both programs are in addition to the $15 million already appropriated under the FY87 continuing resolution, P.L. 99-591; and (2) an additional $35 million each for FY87 and FY88 for Section 8 assistance for the rehabilitation of single room occupancy (SRO) dwellings to be used solely to house the homeless.

• Authorizations, with regard to HHS, for (1) $50 million in FY87 and $30 million in FY88 for new grants to provide outpatient health care to the homeless; (2) $35 million in FY87 and such sums as may be necessary in FY88 for new state block grants to provide outpatient mental health services to the homeless chronically mentally ill; (3) $10 million in FY87 for new alcohol and drug abuse treatment demonstration projects for the homeless to be conducted by community-based public and nonprofit entities; and (4) $40 million for each of FY87 and FY88 for emergency community services grants for the homeless under the community services block grant program.

• Authorizations, with regard to the Department of Education, for (1) $7.5 million in FY87 and $10 million in FY88 for new state grants to develop literacy programs for homeless adults; (2) $5 million for each of FY87 and FY88 for state grants to establish an Office of Coordinator of Education of Homeless Children and Youth in each state to ensure that homeless children have access to public education; and (3) $2.5 million in FY88 for new grants to state and local education agencies for exemplary programs that successfully address the needs of homeless elementary and secondary school students.

• With regard to the Department of Agriculture, the bill will, among other things, (1) allow related families with children who live together to be treated as separate households for the purpose of obtaining food stamps, and (2) prohibit third-party payments on behalf of households residing in temporary shelter that lack adequate cooking facilities from being counted as income for the purpose of obtaining food stamps, thereby increasing benefits for those in certain welfare hotels.

B

The Methodology of Counting the Homeless

Charles D. Cowan, William R. Breakey, and Pamela J. Fischer

Although there has been great interest in the number of homeless Americans in the past decade, few rigorously designed censuses of homeless populations have been mounted. When counts have been attempted, they have been local in scope, and problems with the enumeration methods have not been widely discussed.

The impetus for determining the number of homeless people results largely from increased interest in the projection of service needs and the distribution of resources for the homeless. For example, the U.S. Department of Housing and Urban Development has conducted its own research on the need for emergency shelters; the National Institute for Mental Health administers a number of service programs and has funded several research studies on the demand for services by the homeless; and P.L.'s 98-151 and 98-181 charged the Emergency Food and Shelter National Board with the quick distribution of $40 million to supplement and extend emergency food and shelter services nationwide. In this last case, the distribution of the funds was determined by considering both the overall unemployment rate for an area and the total number of unemployed people within a civil jurisdiction. Although the Emergency Food and Shelter National Board recognizes that "unemployment rates and numbers are not a totally valid surrogate for need or poverty" (1983),

Charles D. Cowan is chief statistician, Center for Education Statistics, U.S. Department of Education. William R. Breakey is director of the Community Psychiatry Program, Department of Psychiatry and Behavioral Sciences, The Johns Hopkins Medical Institutions. Pamela J. Fischer is assistant professor, Department of Psychiatry and Behavioral Sciences, The Johns Hopkins Medical Institutions.

they could find no other data "which were current, uniform and available within the time frame."

Counting the homeless population is extremely difficult because of the lack of a clear definition of homelessness, the mobility of the population, and the cyclical nature of homelessness for many individuals. In addition, homeless people are often reluctant to be interviewed, and many of them remain invisible even to the most diligent of researchers. There is no uniform method for counting the homeless, and very few good studies have been done. Three approaches have been used: indirect estimation, single-contact censuses, and capture-recapture studies. Each method, while offering some benefits, suffers from certain technical inadequacies.

INDIRECT ESTIMATION

The indirect method involves eliciting information from knowledgeable sources, or key informants, about the number of homeless people in an area or the number receiving services, including tallies of the number of people using shelters and other services and estimates of the number of people turned away or otherwise not receiving services. This type of study requires that each of the informants must define "homeless" according to standard criteria and report the number of homeless people encountered over the same period and that the service agencies must be exhaustively surveyed. Because different agencies or groups provide services for the same set of people, some allowance has to be made for double (or multiple) counting of individuals. Unduplication is extremely difficult and requires detailed knowledge of the area and the services under study.

The great advantage of indirect estimation is that it is the most economical method. Data collection in this type of study can be done by telephone or by letter with staff in service agencies and local government bureaus. In addition, publications and service reports that can be used as a base for the counts are often available from the agencies and bureaus. The major disadvantage of this method is its tendency to produce inflated estimates due to duplication. The necessity of reliance on the advice of key informants whose perceptions of the size and nature of the homeless population are biased by their own particular set of experiences and who may be unaware of the extent of the overlap in service utilization may also badly skew that population estimate.

Two much-quoted national studies have reported widely divergent estimates of the national homeless population as determined by indirect estimation techniques. Hombs and Snyder (1982) reported that "in 1980 . . . we concluded that approximately 1 percent of the population, or 2.2 million people, lacked shelter. We arrived at that conclusion on the basis of information received from more than 100 agencies and organizations in 25 cities and states. . . . It is as accurate an estimate as anyone in the country could offer, yet it lacks absolute statistical certainty." This number, despite the flaws inherent in trying to obtain a national estimate from such a small and disparate sample, was for some time the only number available nationally and so attained a certain level of currency.

The second national study, conducted by the U.S. Department of Housing and Urban Development (HUD) (Bobo, 1984), also used the indirect method. Five hundred knowledgeable observers were contacted to obtain local estimates of the number of homeless people in a sample of 60 urban areas. In addition, HUD researchers spoke with 184 shelter managers in a separate random sample of shelters, visited 10 metropolitan areas, and interviewed officials in all 50 states. The HUD report estimated that there were from 250,000 to 300,000 homeless people in the United States.

There were several major flaws in the design and conduct of the HUD research. The first problem was that the contacts made in each of the 60 metropolitan areas were done by "snowball sampling," in which the interviewers first contacted sample units (shelters) that were known to them, and then used the information provided by shelter operators and other knowledgeable people to get names of other shelters or locations not on the initial list. Repetition of this technique should eventually lead to a complete list of all shelters, but several interactions are needed to be certain that the list is complete. Furthermore, this method leads to a different probability of contact for each unit in the population, since the probability is a function of how frequently the shelter is mentioned.

Another problem is the lack of uniformity of response or coverage from the 60 metropolitan areas included in the survey. Many advocates and others deal only with homeless people in their own immediate area, and may have no direct experience with homeless people in other parts of the metropolitan area or a good measure of how much movement there is between areas within the city. Obtaining estimates from people who have studied the homeless population for a whole city may be no better, since their methodologies and definitions vary. The city of Baltimore provides an example, where estimates of the number of homeless people there have ranged from 2,000 to 15,000 (Baltimore City Council, 1983; Health and Welfare Council of Central Maryland, 1983, 1986). Other cities have similar ranges, depending on how the research was done. Aggregating these numbers for 60 metropolitan areas and then weighting the numbers up to the national level may only be expected to produce estimates with larger meaningless ranges.

Applebaum (1986) points out that another problem with the HUD study is that it used population data for Rand McNally metropolitan areas

(RMAs), which include but are much larger than the cities named in the survey. HUD asked respondents about the numbers of homeless estimated for the cities, but applied the reported homeless counts to the whole RMAs. This would lead to an underestimate of the number of homeless in the entire RMA; summing these estimates and weighting them up by the ratio of the U.S. population to the population of the sample RMAs would lead to an underestimate of the size of the homeless population for the entire country.

Finally, many local studies, including some of those incorporated into the HUD (Bobo, 1984) and Hombs and Snyder (1982) estimates, fail to distinguish between "point" estimates, which deal with the number of homeless on a particular day, and "period" estimates, which attempt to give a measure of the numbers of homeless over a period such as a year. The problems in deriving accurate period estimates are much more complex than those in deriving point estimates; estimates of the two types should never be combined.

A good example of an indirect count conducted at the state level is that by the Health and Welfare Council of Central Maryland (1986). A list was developed of all shelter providers in the state, and data were collected from each one regarding the numbers of people sheltered on specific nights throughout the year. Where shelter providers did not keep precise records, they were asked to estimate as closely as possible. In this way an estimate of the number of sheltered homeless people was developed. Estimating the number of homeless people not sheltered presented greater problems. Here again, the investigators asked the informed service providers and other concerned agencies to estimate how many people in their jurisdictions were homeless but not in shelters on given nights. The responses provided very wide ranges of estimates, so the investigators devised weighting systems to be applied to the different counties depending on their levels of economic development and organization. They also employed expert informants to estimate the proportions of homeless people who may not ever come in contact with shelter providers and thus would not even be included in the unsheltered estimate. They developed adjustment factors based on these estimates, despite the fact that there was little unanimity as to the size of this hidden population. They expressed the view that their estimates probably were very conservative. In this way, they concluded that on an average night in 1985, 1,000 homeless people were sheltered in Maryland and that there were an additional 1,900 unserved homeless people. Of this total population of 2,900, 1,160 were in the city of Baltimore; the remainder were distributed throughout the state.

The report briefly mentioned another figure: 28,038 people "reported sheltered during Fiscal Year 1985." The report was careful to point out that this figure is not based on unduplicated data, but on reports from shelter providers about annual volumes of service. The wide difference between this number and the one-night estimate illustrates the hazards of accepting service provider data without very careful consideration of how the data were obtained or whether they represented point or period estimates.

Another statewide indirect count was that done by the Department of Social Services in New York State in 1984 (New York State Department of Social Services, 1984). One thousand agencies were contacted to ascertain whether they were shelter providers. Two hundred and fifty shelter providers were finally identified from this list. Data from these providers led to an estimate of 20,210 single persons and family members as the average nightly sheltered population. In order to allow for the numbers of homeless people outside the shelter system, they used ratios of shelter:street populations derived from studies in Boston and Pittsburgh to arrive at a total statewide estimate of 50,362. The authors acknowledge that the use of these ratios, derived from estimates obtained by different methods in very different settings, is questionable. Additional data supplied by the shelter providers as well as by hospitals, police departments, and other informants supplemented the counts, to give more information on the composition of the homeless population.

SINGLE-CONTACT CENSUSES

The single-contact census is a technique that has been used in cities to make estimates of the size of their homeless populations. The census is usually taken by teams of individuals in a clearly defined area where preliminary studies suggest that the largest proportion of the homeless population can be found. A screening questionnaire, or, at the very least, instructions for selecting individuals to approach, are given to the teams conducting the census. Under optimum conditions the census should be conducted in a single day, preferably during a time of day when the homeless people are most likely to be stationary, such as late at night. However, for practical reasons, many censuses of this type are conducted over a short period of time with some mechanism for recognizing and eliminating duplications.

The advantages of a single-contact census are twofold: It provides for direct contact, even if only by observation so that the possibility of counting individuals more than once is reduced, and there is greater assurance that the people contacted fit the study's definition of homelessness. In addition, demographics and other information can be obtained that may be crucial to determining the type and level of services that need to be provided for this population.

There are also two primary disadvantages of a single-contact census. The census provides a cross-sectional view of the population at a single point in time, but because the homeless population appears to be in a constant state of flux (Bachrach, 1984; Bassuk, 1984; Lamb, 1984; Fischer and Breakey, 1986), it is out of date almost immediately after it is taken. Moreover, it may poorly represent the true homeless population if taken at the wrong time. If, for example, the number of homeless people on the streets is reduced on the few days after welfare or various types of social assistance payments become available, the number of homeless people may be underestimated.

Another disadvantage of a single-contact census is that it is expensive relative to indirect estimation. It is necessary to use a team of enumerators to comb areas of the city where data are being collected. For reasons of safety, workers are usually deployed in teams of at least two people who are often accompanied by off-duty police officers. Staffing costs are thus quite high.

An excellent single-contact census of the urban homeless was conducted in Washington, D.C., by the Center for Applied Research and Urban Policy of the University of the District of Columbia (Robinson, 1985). The study was carefully designed, and its techniques and assumptions are carefully documented. The investigators counted all the residents of the various shelters in Washington on a specific night, July 31, 1985, and obtained counts of homeless people in hospitals and other institutions. They supplemented this with a search of other places on the streets where people may be found at night. The city was divided into 20 count areas, with an enumerating team assigned to each area. The enumerators worked in pairs; each pair included a research assistant and a person experienced in working with the homeless. The investigators recognized that a certain number of homeless people would fail to be counted either because their appearance was unremarkable or because they chose concealed locations in which to sleep. An intensive search was therefore made in one area of the city with an augmented team that included a police officer to judge to what extent the less intensive counts may have failed to find homeless individuals who were hidden from view. A series of five estimates were made, based on the direct counts and including corrections for the two sources of error, underenumeration because people were not identified as homeless and underenumeration because people were actively avoiding being counted. The estimates ranged from 4,347 to 7,152, with the highest value being 64 percent larger than the lowest value.

Other recent single-count censuses have been conducted in a number of cities by surveying homeless people at sites that provide services, such as shelters, soup kitchens, and social service departments (Brown et al., 1983; Chaiklin, 1983; McGerigle and Lauriat, 1983). However, with survey sites of this sort there is an increased risk of duplication. This risk can be minimized by including brief screening questions and by restricting the data collection activities to a relatively short period. Surveys at sites that provide services can also have the problem of being dependent on agency personnel who may abandon or ignore the data collection because it interferes with their provision of services.

Multiple-count studies expand on the single-count methodology by conducting counts at two or more points in time. These studies are designed so that the counts are combined to produce a single estimate. Such studies provide additional information about changes in the population over time, documenting seasonal and other variations.

A recent study of this type was conducted in Chicago in 1985 and 1986, by Rossi and colleagues (1986). First, all homeless people in shelters were counted. Then, in order to estimate the number of street people, a survey design was developed to sample blocks in the city where homeless people were expected to concentrate according to information obtained from police and other informants. These blocks were then surveyed by research workers accompanied by police officers. This process was repeated 6 months later. Despite much effort, the yield of homeless people on the streets that were counted by this technique was very low, with only 22 being identified on the first occasion and 28 on the second. Based on these institutional and street samples, estimates were derived for the total homeless population of Chicago. The estimates, 5,907 on the first occasion and 3,719 on the second, were widely criticized by people familiar with homelessness in Chicago as being much too low. Previous estimates, derived by indirect methods, ranged from 12,000 to 25,000 (Chicago Department of Human Services, 1983). Another finding that casts doubt on the conclusions of this study is that no children were included in the counts of people on the streets, though families with small children are believed to make up as much as 40 percent of Chicago's homeless population (U.S. Conference of Mayors, 1986). Applebaum (1986) points out that many of the homeless people contacted on the streets may have denied that they were homeless. It is amazing that in a sample of blocks identified as likely places to encounter the homeless, only 22 of 318 individuals encountered would be homeless in phase I of the study, and only 28 of 289 would be homeless in phase II. Rossi and associates (1986) admitted that even when the police officers who accompanied the interviewers were not immediately introduced, subjects were always able to identify them as police officers, and therefore, they started the interaction on a negative note. In addition, the teams conducted preliminary observations of the blocks before any formal screening started, thereby tipping off a naturally suspicious population to their presence.

Having two counts enabled the investigators to comment on the differences in the findings obtained in October 1985 compared with those obtained in March 1986. In view of the methodological problems described above, however, the validity of these conclusions must be held in question.

Another multiple-count census was done in Nashville (Wiegard, 1985), where the homeless were counted on four separate occasions (the first day of each season) over the course of a year. Because Nashville is a much smaller city, the elaborate sampling frame used in the Chicago study was not needed and the entire downtown area could be surveyed during a single night. Demographic distributions observed at different times were used to draw conclusions about the changing nature of the homeless population in Nashville. The study concluded that although the estimated numbers of homeless people varied relatively little, from 689 to 836, the ratios of homeless found in shelters compared with the homeless found on the streets varied with the seasons. During the winter the ratio was found to be 25:1, but in the fall the ratio was 5:1.

Such ratios have been a focus of interest in several studies, including the study done for New York State by its Department of Social Services described above. The HUD report used an estimate that the shelter to street ratio was about 1:2 (Bobo, 1984). This estimate was derived from ratios of 100:129 estimated for Boston (Boston Emergency Shelter Commission, 1983), 100:130 for Pittsburgh (Winograd, 1982), and 100:273 for Phoenix (Brown et al., 1983).

Freeman and Hall (1986) attempted to use a ratio of this sort based on a survey of about 500 homeless people in New York City to make generalizations about the national homeless population. Apart from the obvious criticism that there is no logical basis for generalizing from New York City to the country as a whole, the many problems with this study included the local and unusual nature of their survey sample and their failure to take into account the cyclical patterns of homelessness. In attempting to generalize from their ratios to the national level, they based their estimates on the flawed HUD data and failed to take into account the variability of street:shelter ratios described above for various cities. Their conclusions, therefore, must be interpreted with considerable skepticism.

CAPTURE-RECAPTURE METHODS

Capture-recapture methods go beyond multiple-count methods by matching data on individuals observed at two or more points in time. They thus permit certain conclusions about the movement of individuals in and out of the population, as well as statistics about the population from which the sample was drawn. Capture-recapture techniques involve matching observations of individuals made at each of two or more data collection periods. In wildlife populations, for which this technique was developed, captured animals were tagged for ready identification on recapture. Matching of homeless individuals is achieved by using a combination of name, Social Security number, birth date, sex, race, and other unique identifiers. In matching subjects from the first observation to the second, the resulting data can be tabulated as shown in Table B-1.

The values in Table B-1 represent counts of people observed at different times: N_1 represents the count of those obtained during the first data collection period, N_2 represents the count of those obtained during the second data collection period, and M represents the number matched, that is, the number observed both times. The only number missing from Table B-1 that cannot be easily calculated by subtraction is the number of people in the population not observed in either the first or second period.

Two estimates of the number of homeless people in an area are possible from Table B-1. The first assumes that the census was complete and that the missing cell (not observed in either period) actually should have an entry of one. This estimate of the total number of homeless would be calculated as $N_1 + N_2 - M$ (Equation B-1). This estimate would then be merely a lower bound to the actual number of homeless, since in reality no census is complete and there are hidden homeless who remain uncounted no matter how strenuous an effort is made.

A second estimate can be calculated from Table B-1 that does not assume that there are no hidden homeless, and this is the estimate by the capture-recapture method. This assumes that each data collection is imperfect, that there is some probability at each data collection that individuals will be missed, and that consequently there is some (unknown) probability that individuals will be missed both times. The estimate of the total number of homeless from a capture-recapture study can be calculated from the formula $(N_1 \times N_1)/M$ (Equation B-2). Capture-recapture estimates have been used for biometric applications for several

TABLE B-1   Observation of the Homeless in
Two Periods of Time

First Period of Time	Second Period of Time		Total
	Matched	Not Matched	
Matched	M		N_1
Not matched			
Total count	N_2		

hundred years, chiefly in making estimates of the size of wildlife populations, and the basic estimator (Equation B-2) has been rederived in several different contexts. One of the earliest use of capture-recapture techniques for human populations was for the evaluation of the completeness of birth and death records (Chandrasekar and Deming, 1949). The most common application currently is for the evaluation of population and agriculture censuses (Cowan et al., 1986). Also called dual-system estimation in this context, evaluations of censuses by capture-recapture studies have been conducted in the United States, Paraguay, Bangladesh, India, and other countries. The evaluation of the census and use of the capture-recapture method in Somalia is of particular interest, since 60 percent of that country's population is nomadic and, in this respect, is similar to a homeless population. Additional information on a population can be obtained from making more than two observations. In recent years, maximum likelihood techniques have been used to derive estimates for use in studies involving several sampling periods (Bishop et al., 1976).

There are two studies of homeless populations that make use of capture-recapture techniques. The first was a study of the number of homeless men in Sydney, Australia (Darcy and Jones, 1975). In that study of homeless men, three 1-day censuses were conducted at 25 locations including shelters, hospitals, clinics, and a jail, on June 30, 1971; October 13, 1971; and March 8, 1972. Using Equation B-2, three estimates of the number of homeless men were obtained by comparing the three sets of data, two at a time, with the following results: June to October, 3,025; June to March, 4,119; and October to March, 3,322. The authors used a related technique that makes use of information from all three data sets to yield an overall estimate of the number of homeless men in Sydney (3,200). They also estimated the average "birth" and "death" rates for men entering and leaving the homeless population to be 21 and 5 percent, respectively, indicating that the homeless population was increasing over the period of the study.

It should be noted from the estimates presented above that the longer the interval between counts, the higher the estimate. The authors noted that the intervals between censuses were sufficiently long to allow entry and exit from the homeless population, through moving in and out of Sydney, deaths, and so on, so that the numbers of matches were reduced. If shorter time intervals had been used, it might be supposed that the estimates would have been lower.

The other study that used the capture-recapture method was conducted in Baltimore in 1985 and 1986 (Cowan et al., 1986). Four pairs of dates were chosen in August and November 1985 and in February and May 1986 to reflect the four seasons; each pair was used for a capture-recapture estimate. Data were entered on separate computer files for the eight counts, and a computer program was written to match individuals between counts. Each of the four pairs of counts permitted a capture-recapture estimate of the total number of potential shelter users in the city on an average night in that month. The results indicated that the number of people in the shelter-using population did not vary significantly across the seasons, ranging from 874 to 1,022. The counts also showed that on all eight nights the shelter beds in the city were filled close to capacity. From the computer lists it was possible to create a master file of individuals observed at any of the eight sampling periods, including demographic information and a record of sample in which they were included. The master file included 2,102 people, of whom 66 percent were men and 34 percent were women. Analysis of the patterns of recurrence of individuals in successive samples provided information on the dynamics of people entering and leaving the homeless population.

In order to make an estimate of the proportion of homeless people who do not use the shelter system, a street survey was conducted in December 1986. People were questioned very briefly in places where homeless people congregate, but do not sleep, such as soup kitchens, day shelters, or on the streets. The brief questionnaire asked whether they had a place to live, and if not, did they use the shelter system, and if so, when was the most recent occasion. This information was then used to supplement the capture-recapture estimates. It was found that about three-quarters of those questioned were potential shelter users. Taking this into account, the capture-recapture estimates from this study provided estimates that were very compatible with those obtained by the indirect survey method in the Health and Welfare Council of Central Maryland (1986) study described above, in which the total number estimated for Baltimore was 1,160 and the sex ratio was 64 percent male to 36 percent female.

The most important difference between the capture-recapture technique and the two methods described earlier is that the capture-recapture technique is the only one that involves a statistical model to estimate the size of the unseen portion of the population. Single- or multiple-count censuses require some correction or expansion on the counts obtained, to allow for the hidden homeless who are not included in shelter counts, or in the case of the single-contact census, who may not even be picked up in a well-done street census. The correction factors used in most studies did not seem to be calculated under any rigorous statistical procedure but, rather, reflected the ratio the researchers wanted to obtain.

A statistical model involves a number of assumptions about factors that affect or, perhaps more important, that do not affect the data collection process. The most important assumptions in the capture-recapture method are listed below:

1. Clear definitions: Homeless people can be accurately identified.

2. Homogeneous observation probabilities: Each person has the same chance of being observed in a specific period.

3. Stability: The size and nature of the population does not change during the observation period.

4. Stationarity: The population does not move in or out of the study area during the observation period.

5. Independent captures: For the periods, the order interaction term (however defined) is zero; that is, even though a homeless person was observed at one period, it does not affect the probability that the person will be observed on subsequent occasions.

6. Data correctness: The information collected is accurate.

7. Complete response: Individuals or informants provide information that is complete enough to permit matching.

8. Matching correctness: Data records for the same individuals can be linked between observation periods.

9. Single observations: Individuals are observed only once at each data collection.

10. Known externalities: Factors that affect the data collection are known and can be accounted for, such as weather conditions and receipt of welfare checks.

Violations of these assumptions invalidate the model, causing the results to be biased (Cowan, 1982, 1984). More complex models allow for all exigencies, but more complex models require more data and may be impractical.

DISCUSSION

Although the existence of a sizable homeless population is beyond doubt and there is a consensus among knowledgeable people that the extent of the problem has been increasing in recent years, the ever-changing and fluid nature of the homeless population presents great methodological challenges in obtaining an accurate measure of its size. A review of the methods for estimating the number of homeless people indicates that great caution should be exercised in interpreting any of the available data. Each of the methods that has been used has inherent biases. There is no national estimate that is based on a sound methodology and that is agreed to be accurate. Estimates prepared for individual communities or cities may be more accurate, but here also, careful scrutiny of methodology is required to assess such data adequately.

In order to advance research in this area, developmental work is needed in three specific areas:

1. Definitions must be developed concerning who is considered homeless. Agreement on a definition is vital if valid comparisons between studies are to be made. Subgroups, such as homeless families, should also be defined.

2. There is a need for more comparative research to determine better methodologies for studying difficult to find or difficult to enumerate populations. An example would be research in the use of network or multiplicity sampling for making estimates of the size of the homeless population in cities.

3. There is a need for more comprehensive capture-recapture models. Such models would permit data from several sources to be used and adjustments for missing data to be incorporated into the model.

Future research must pay very careful attention to the biases introduced by the different enumeration methods. Research teams must take advantage of the knowledge of people who are familiar with the homeless population in designing data collection techniques and in defining and identifying homeless people. Even with careful attention to methodological issues, it may not be practical or possible to develop a valid national estimate of the total number of homeless people. If, however, studies are carried out in cities and communities across the country using clear definitions and clearly defined methods, a composite picture may be built that will ultimately be more informative.

REFERENCES

Applebaum, R. P. 1986. Counting the homeless. Paper prepared for the George Washington University Conference on Homelessness.

Bachrach, L. L. 1984. The homeless mentally ill and mental health services: An analytic review of the literature. In The Homeless Mentally Ill, H. R. Lamb, ed. Washington, D.C.: American Psychiatric Association.

Baltimore City Council. 1983. Report of the Baltimore City Task Force for the Homeless. Baltimore: Baltimore City Council.

Bassuk, E. L. 1984. The homeless problem. Scientific American 251(1):40–45.

Bishop, Y. M. M., S. E. Feinberg, and P. W. Holland. 1976. Discrete Multivariate Analysis. Cambridge, Mass.: MIT Press.

Bobo, B. F. 1984. A Report to the Secretary on the Homeless and Emergency Shelters. Washington, D.C.: U.S. Department of Housing and Urban Development.

Boston Emergency Shelter Commission. 1983. The October Project: Seeing the Obvious Problem. Boston: Boston Emergency Shelter Commission.

Brown, C., S. McFarlane, R. Paredes, and L. Stark. 1983. The Homeless of Phoenix: Who Are They and What Should Be Done? Phoenix, Ariz.: Phoenix South Community Mental Health Center.

Chaiklin, H. 1983. The service needs of soup kitchen users. Baltimore: School of Social Work and Community Planning, University of Maryland. (Unpublished.)

Chandrasekar, C., and W. E. Deming. 1949. On a method of estimating birth and death rates and the extent of registration. Journal of the American Statistical Association 44:101–115.

Chicago Department of Human Services. 1983. Homelessness in Chicago. Chicago: Chicago Department of Human Services.

Cowan, C. D. 1982. Modifications to capture-recapture estimation in the presence of errors in the data. Paper presented at the meetings of the American Statistical Association, Biometrics Section, Cincinnati.

Cowan, C. D. 1984. The Effects of Misclassification on Estimates from the Capture-Recapture Studies. Unpublished Ph.D. dissertation. The George Washington University, Washington, D.C..

Cowan, C. D., W. R. Breakey, and P. J. Fischer. 1986. The methodology of counting the homeless. In Proceedings of the American Statistical Association, Survey Research Methods Section. Alexandria, Va.: American Statistical Association.

Cowan, C. D., R. J. Magnani, P. P. Biemer, and A. G. Turner. 1985. Evaluating Censuses of Population and Housing. Washington, D.C.: Bureau of the Census.

Darcy, L., and D. L. Jones. 1975. The size of the homeless men population of Sydney. Australian Journal of Social Issues 10:208–215.

Emergency Food and Shelter National Board. 1983. Program Description. A board established by Congress and the United Way. Alexandria, Va.: United Way of America.

Fischer, P. J., and W. R. Breakey. 1986. Homelessness and mental health: An overview. International Journal of Mental Health 14(4):6–41.

Freeman, R. B., and B. Hall. 1986. Permanent Homelessness in America: Working paper no. 2013. Cambridge, Mass.: National Bureau of Economic Analysis.

Health and Welfare Council of Central Maryland. 1983. A Report to the Greater Baltimore Shelter Network on Homelessness in Central Maryland. Baltimore: Health and Welfare Council of Central Maryland.

Health and Welfare Council of Central Maryland. 1986. Where Do You Go from Nowhere? Homelessness in Maryland. Baltimore: Maryland Department of Human Resources.

Hombs, M. E., and M. Snyder. 1982. Homelessness in America: A Forced March to Nowhere. Washington, D.C.: Community for Creative Nonviolence.

Lamb, H. R., ed. 1984. The Homeless Mentally Ill. Washington, D.C.: The American Psychiatric Association.

McGerigle, P., and A. S. Lauriat. 1983. More Than Shelter: A Community Response to Homelessness. Boston: United Community Planning Corporation.

New York State Department of Social Services. 1984. Homelessness in New York State: A Report to the Governor and the Legislature. New York: New York State Department of Social Services.

Robinson, F. G. 1985. Homeless People in the Nation's Capital. Washington, D.C.: Center for Applied Research and Urban Policy, University of the District of Columbia.

Rossi, P. H., G. A. Fisher, and G. Willis. 1986. The Condition of the Homeless in Chicago. A report prepared by the Social and Demographic Research Institute, University of Massachusetts at Amherst, and the National Opinion Research Center, University of Chicago.

U.S. Conference of Mayors. 1986. The Continued Growth of Hunger, Homelessness and Poverty in America's Cities: 1986. A 25-City Survey. Washington, D.C.: U.S. Conference of Mayors.

Wiegard, R. B. 1985. Counting the homeless. American Demographics 7(12):34–37.

Winograd, K. 1982. Street People and Other Homeless: A Pittsburgh Study. Pittsburgh: The Emergency Shelter Task Force.

C The Rural Homeless

Larry T. Patton

Homelessness is a reality for a growing number of rural Americans. This situation has received little notice, as media and research attention has focused on the highly visible problem of the urban homeless. This lack of public recognition is hardly surprising. Rural residents have a long tradition of preferring self-help and reliance on relatives, friends, and neighbors to taxpayer-supported programs, which has effectively disguised the magnitude of the problem of rural homelessness. Some would even argue that while private, voluntary action was meeting the need, the policy implications of ignoring the rural homeless were minimal.

The situation appears to be changing, however. There are growing indications that some rural communities can no longer shoulder the burden alone. Informal community support networks are being over-whelmed by the severity and duration of the rural economic crisis. Farm communities, in particular, are experiencing an erosion of the old rural ethic that "we take care of our own," a development that appears to be independent of the rural economic crisis.

At this point, there are no answers to many questions central to the public policy debate: issues of definition, the prevalence of rural home-lessness, changes in its incidence, and similarities and differences between rural and urban homeless populations. Unfortunately, this appendix cannot authoritatively resolve these questions; that will require substantial additional field research. The discussion presented here relies instead on a review of the meager available research, a special survey conducted

Larry T. Patton is a Washington, D.C.-based consultant specializing in health and welfare policy and rural issues.

by the U.S. Department of Health and Human Services (HHS) of its community health center grantees, and two site visits—to the Black Belt counties of Alabama and Mississippi and the farm regions of Minnesota and North Dakota—that were supported by HHS. While broad generalizations cannot be drawn from the site visits, they proved particularly useful in providing sharply contrasting views of homelessness.

This appendix first examines the nature and causes of homelessness in rural areas. The structural transformation now under way in the rural economy, the nature of the rural environment, and rural social service networks are briefly reviewed, as is the available evidence regarding the characteristics of the rural homeless.

The remainder of the appendix examines the scanty data on medical care utilization by the homeless. The primary sources of data include a study supported by the National Institute of Mental Health of the homeless in Ohio and the community health center survey and site visits mentioned above.

This appendix offers a number of observations:

• Rural homelessness is essentially an economic problem. The failure of policymakers to appreciate the extent of the rural economic crisis, and the degree to which a majority of rural counties are especially vulnerable, has contributed to the tendency to perceive homelessness exclusively as an urban problem.

• The nature of rural communities obscures the problem of homelessness as well. With the exception of larger, more urbanized cities, rural communities seldom have in place a formal social service network that would permit the transient homeless to gather or be counted. In fact, they are often met with hostility and suspicion by community residents.

• The willingness of neighbors to "take care of their own," shuttling the economically distressed family from neighbor to neighbor, has been a major factor leading to underestimates of the rural homeless. The site visits also highlighted the significant private efforts being made by philanthropic and religious organizations to assist the homeless.

• The duration and the pervasiveness of the economic crisis may increase the public burden of rural homelessness. An important finding in farming communities is the growing evidence that those in economic distress can no longer rely on their neighbors for help.

• The rural homeless appear to be slightly younger than their urban counterparts and more likely to be living in intact, two-parent families in which both parents were recently employed before being forced into poverty and homelessness.

• The ability to access medical care in times of emergency appears adequate, but this finding is tentative at best. There are few data on the homeless living in the sparsely populated areas where provider shortages would be more common.

• Routine or preventive care is used little, if at all, which is similar to the case for the urban homeless. The high prevalence of chronic disease in the rural population and the high rates of malnutrition, dental disease, and environmental hazards (poor sanitation, inadequate and dangerous housing, and contaminated water supplies) suggest the importance of access to such care.

• There is a great need to better utilize the existing delivery systems, such as community, rural, and migrant health care centers, to address the medical care needs of the rural homeless.

A final point deserves to be mentioned: the issue of relative burden. Compared to urban America, there are great differences in the scale, density, and resource base of rural communities that severely limit the ability of these communities to assist individuals in economic distress. That perspective is essential to keep in mind as we develop better estimates of the relative distribution of the homeless in rural and urban communities. Even relatively low numbers of homeless individuals and families can easily overwhelm a rural community's resources.

THE RURAL ECONOMIC CRISIS

Parts of rural America are facing their worst economic crisis since the Great Depression. In the last few years, the rural economy has been dealt a series of economic setbacks.

• Farm foreclosures have been taking place at a staggering rate: 650,000 foreclosures have occurred since 1981 and another 2,000 farmers give up farming each week.

• Low-wage, labor-intensive rural manufacturing has lost over half a million jobs since 1981 as a result of foreign competition.

• Timber, mining, petroleum, and other energy industries experienced severe downturns as energy prices tumbled (Sinclair, 1987; Brown and Deavers, no date).

The secondary effects have been just as severe. It is estimated that one business fails for each six to seven farms lost to foreclosure (Ranney, 1986); in fact, in 1985, 130 banks closed, the highest number in any year since the Great Depression (U.S. Congress, Senate, Committee on Governmental Affairs, 1986). The rural unemployment rate now consistently exceeds the urban unemployment rate, a reversal of the historical trend. In addition, the rural poverty rate approached the 20 percent mark, the highest level in two decades (Brown and Deavers, no date).

Yet the impact of these economic changes on rural counties has been uneven: Some rural counties have experienced few repercussions from the worsening economic climate; others have been devastated. Two aspects of the rural economy are useful in identifying those rural counties most at risk.

First, most rural counties have never successfully diversified their economic base. As a result, the economies of two out of every three nonmetropolitan counties are dominated by a single industry. In 1985, of the 2,443 nonmetropolitan counties, 29 percent (702 counties) were primarily dependent on agriculture, 28 percent (678 counties) were manufacturing dependent, and 8 percent (200 counties) were mining dependent (Brown and Deavers, no date).* All of these industries are in financial distress.

Second, while poverty has left few rural counties untouched, rural poverty has always been extremely concentrated. Two-thirds of the rural poor reside in the southeastern states, as do 93 percent of rural blacks (Ghelfi, 1986; National Association of Community Health Centers, 1987). Of the 231 counties that have ranked in the bottom fifth of income for the past 30 years, all but 18 are located in the southeastern United States. In fact, four states (Georgia, Kentucky, Mississippi, and Tennessee) each had more than 20 such counties. The 18 persistently poor counties outside the South were all minority dominated (Hoppe, 1985).

Counties whose economies are dominated by a single industry in distress—particularly those plagued by persistent poverty—offer displaced workers few job alternatives. Unfortunately, there is little basis on which to predict whether rural displaced workers will migrate to metropolitan areas, where some may contribute to the urban homeless problem, or remain in rural areas. While there is now under way a net migration away from rural areas (Sinclair, 1987), migration clearly works in both directions. Migrant laborers; those alienated from urban life; unsuccessful job seekers in urban areas returning to their families; and even those accidentally stranded in their job searches due to emotional, financial, or physical collapse all contribute to migration into rural areas (Frank and Streeter, 1987). In addition, the rapid rise in the poverty and unemployment rates in rural areas demonstrates that many rural residents have chosen to remain, despite the low probability of finding alternative employment above the minimum wage.

*A county is viewed as being dependent on a specific industry when the weighted average annual income of the industry accounts for 20 percent or more of weighted annual total labor and proprietor income, according to Brown and Deavers (no date).

DEFINING RURAL HOMELESSNESS

The impediments to establishing a clear-cut definition of homelessness in urban areas are only exacerbated in rural America. Clearly, all displaced workers or farmers do not always join the ranks of the homeless; many do not even make it into the official unemployment count.

How then do we define those who are homeless in rural areas? Do we include those in substandard housing? How do we treat those living with friends and relatives? Do we exclude those who pay nominal rents? At what point does a temporary housing arrangement become permanent? The following case highlights this dilemma:

Family of three (elderly woman, adult daughter, infant grandchild) living in two-room shack (family home for over 20 years on relatives' property in rural area); approximate dimensions, 12 by 20 feet. No electricity, water, or septic tank. Shack is located in area of water runoff and floor is wet most of the year. (Household) head receives disability (Supplemental Security Income), adult woman works minimum-wage job. Rent is $40/month. Water is carried one-half mile from church spigot; has privy. Has been on waiting list 2 years for Section 8 (housing); list is 4 years long. House cannot be winterized due to size and placement of wood stoves, it is felt that making the house weathertight would increase danger of fire. No available affordable housing for this family at this time.

This example was volunteered by a Community Action Agency director as a portrait of their "typical" homelessness case, and it is very compelling.* But elements of this profile are unsettling: Is this family truly homeless? The literature review and the site visits did not provide an operational definition of rural homelessness, but they did provide a general framework for approaching the question.

First, there is little disagreement that those without any form of shelter are homeless; the critical question is the extent to which any definition includes those who are temporarily housed as well. In urban areas, researchers have the option of including selective groups of people with temporary housing, such as the portion of the homeless served by shelters. In truly rural areas, such an option is unavailable because formal services such as shelters are virtually nonexistent; residents who become homeless must rely on friends, neighbors, and relatives for temporary housing.

A relative or friend will often bear the burden alone, initially; later, sharing responsibility by "shuttling the person (or family) along from

---

*This was one Community Action Agency director's response to a survey being conducted by the Housing Assistance Council (1984) of Washington, D.C. The survey was not complete when this report was drafted.

family to family as their 'welcome' is exhausted" (Ohio Department of Mental Health, 1985). Data on rural households suggest that the demands placed on friends and families have escalated rapidly in the 1980s. The Housing Assistance Council, tracking rural household size from 1979 to 1983, found that:

> . . . the increase in rural working poverty over that period was strongly associated with an increase in household size, not by one or two persons, but by three or more persons. Such large increases, we believe, can only be explained by wide-scale doubling up among working poor families. (Wilson, 1983)

While the inclusion of those with temporary housing in rural areas presents serious methodological problems for researchers, the evidence suggests that there are few alternatives to their inclusion; otherwise, similarly situated urban and rural homeless people would be classified differently.

Second, in some cases the homeless pay nominal rents. One source of housing for the homeless is substandard, seemingly abandoned housing stock. In urban areas, much of this property appears to be commercial or owned by absentee landlords, often enabling the homeless to make use of it virtually unnoticed. The site visits conducted by committee members and the author suggested that these types of dwellings are often located on private property that is either occupied by the owner or adjacent to the owner's property. Because of the increased visibility of transients in rural communities, and the proximity of the property's owner, it was not unusual to see nominal rents imposed on those taking refuge in such dwellings.

Finally, for an individual or family to be considered homeless, the housing arrangement must be temporary or unstable; there must be a need to search constantly for more permanent quarters because of the fear of imminent eviction or displacement. The case outlined above lacks this element of instability; it has served as a family dwelling for more than 20 years.

This appendix thus considers individuals or families as homeless if their housing situation is both unstable and temporary (whether it is in a formal shelter, in a makeshift dwelling, or with friends, without regard for the payment of nominal rent) and they lack the resources to secure adequate housing. It is important to reemphasize that the essential criterion is the instability of the housing arrangement; otherwise, we would simply be redefining the nearly 2 million rural poor who live in substandard housing as homeless, which would not be accurate (Housing Assistance Council, 1984). At the same time, individuals or families awaiting certain eviction in the very near future would be categorized as homeless under this definition.

WHO ARE THE RURAL HOMELESS?

It is predictably difficult to answer this question. The rural homeless are more geographically dispersed and the shelter facilities available in rural areas tend to be small, making it difficult for even shelter operators to categorize the population definitively. We will use two approaches to answer this question: The first is a conceptual framework for classifying the rural homeless; next, we will review the Ohio Mental Health study, which, while limited as a single-state case study, provides the only comprehensive statistical comparison of the rural and urban homeless that has been completed to date.

A useful framework developed by Frank and Streeter (1987) suggests that the rural homeless can be categorized into five distinct groups: (1) the traditional homeless, (2) the new poor, (3) the mentally ill, (4) displaced farmers and farm-related workers, and (5) the new hermits.* This grouping can be examined from two perspectives. In comparison with the urban homeless, the latter two groups (displaced farmers and farm-related workers and new hermits) are unique to rural areas. Another perspective is the extent to which these groups reflect the "new" homeless, whose descent into homelessness is of relatively recent origin. That grouping would primarily include the new poor and displaced farmers and farm-related workers.

The Traditional Homeless

These are the street people similar to many of those seen in urban areas, suffering from substance abuse, personal tragedy, or mental or physical disabilities. They have had little recent attachment to the labor force and have trouble maintaining a permanent address or securing employment. They are predominantly single men.

The New Poor

Driven by financial catastrophe, this category has made the largest contribution to the number of rural homeless in recent years. For the most part, they are the working poor or near poor and are two-parent families with children; in most cases, both parents hold part- or full-time jobs. The combination of the recent recessions and the structural transformation of the rural economy often leaves them with few local employment opportunities. As their meager savings are quickly eroded, they

---

*This section is drawn directly from the typology of Frank and Streeter (1987, pp. 39–42).

190   APPENDIX C

are faced with two equally unpalatable alternatives: move in with friends or travel in search of employment.

Those choosing to move on often find free shelter unavailable and are forced to rely on abandoned dwellings, sleeping with the entire family in their vehicles, or, in warmer climates, camping out. A recent study suggests that the homeless are making use of state and federal campground areas (Mariani, 1987). For example, in one Maricopa County, Arizona, campground, over half of the campers were homeless people in search of jobs. For those choosing to move in temporarily with friends, neighbors, or relatives, the hazards are different: Stress often builds quickly in overcrowded quarters and may result in both psychological and physical abuse (Redburn and Buss, 1987).

The Mentally Ill

The number of chronically mentally ill patients in specific rural communities varies significantly. For the most part, they appear to gravitate toward the larger rural communities or towns within close proximity to state mental hospitals. For example, there appeared to be a substantial chronically mentally ill homeless population in the Minnesota-North Dakota shelters, all of which were within close proximity to state mental hospitals. By contrast, the Alabama and Mississippi site visit identified few chronically mentally ill patients.

Displaced Farmers and Farm-Related Workers

The pace of farm foreclosures has resulted in the displacement of large numbers of farmers and farm-related workers. Social workers dealing with farm families argue strongly that farmers face unique stresses as a result of foreclosure. Foreclosure represents the loss of the family home, the farmer's job and primary social network, and the children's inheritance; if the farm has been in the family for several generations, the guilt and self-recrimination are magnified.

When foreclosures are especially numerous in an area, banks and lending institutions often have trouble reselling the farms quickly. As a result, farm families are often permitted to remain as caretakers on a day-to-day basis with eviction quickly following the final sale of the property. From the point of foreclosure, farmers in this unstable and transient position are essentially homeless under our definition.

The site visits confirmed earlier work (Frank and Streeter, 1987) that farmers seldom make use of the available shelters in the larger rural communities; anecdotal evidence suggests that they rely on friends or relatives in other parts of the county or neighboring counties for temporary housing. Service providers consistently agreed that this population is greatly in need: marriages dissolve; generations are divided; family abuse rates are up; and alcoholism, stress, depression, and suicide attempts are on the rise (Wall, 1985; Heffernen and Heffernen, 1986).

This group also includes migrant and seasonal farm workers whose housing, health care, and social service needs have never been adequately met by the existing delivery systems, even in the best of times.

The New Hermits

There is a new group of homeless that is small in number. They have sought refuge in the mountains of Arkansas, Oregon, Washington, and West Virginia. Some are "survivalists," Vietnam veterans, "back-to-the-landers," and others who are isolated from mainstream American society.

There are few data about these individuals and little understanding of whether their homelessness is by choice or economic necessity.

THE OHIO STUDY

Statistical data on the rural homeless have not been collected on the national level. The most exhaustive and authoritative effort to date was the 1985 Ohio Mental Health Study (Ohio Department of Mental Health, 1985).* Because the researchers conducted extensive interviews with 790 urban and 189 nonurban homeless people, their survey provides the most extensive data base available on the demographics of the rural homeless and the ways in which they are both similar and different from their urban counterparts.

These data cannot be generalized to the nation. It is, after all, a case study of one state. Despite that limitation, the Ohio study data provide a rich source of information for developing a preliminary sense of the rural homeless.

In categorizing their data, the Ohio researchers looked at three types of counties: urban, rural, and mixed (rural counties adjacent to urban areas). In preparing their summary tables, some of which are reproduced here, most of the data are consolidated into two categories: urban and nonurban (which includes both the rural and mixed counties). When this combination distorts the analysis, the data will be disaggregated. All of the tables in this section have been reproduced from the Ohio study's final reports, although evidence from other studies and the interviews conducted for this paper will also be cited.

---

*The tables and analysis are drawn directly from the chapter on urban/nonurban comparisons, Ohio Department of Mental Health (1985, p. 53).

Demographics

Table C-1 provides a summary comparison of the demographics of the urban and nonurban populations interviewed by the Ohio research team. A few highlights are given below.

Sex and Marital Status

Women constitute a much higher proportion of the rural homeless population (32.3 versus 15.8 percent of the urban homeless), a fact that is partly explained by the much higher percentage of rural homeless who are married (18.5 percent of the rural homeless versus 6.7 percent of the urban homeless).

Ethnicity

Ethnicity reflects the demographics of the state and is representative of many Midwestern states, which do not have significant minority populations other than blacks (e.g., Hispanics or Indians).

Age

On average, the rural homeless are a slightly younger population, with 72 percent being under age 40 (versus 60 percent of the urban homeless that are under age 40). These results are parallel to those of a study in Vermont, in which it was found that most homeless are in their early 30s

TABLE C-1   Demographic Comparison of Urban and Nonurban Counties (Ohio Data)

Characteristic	Urban No.	Urban Percent	Nonurban No.	Nonurban Percent	Total No.	Total Percent
Sex						
Male	665	84.2	128	67.7	793	81.0
Female	125	15.8	61	32.3	186	19.0
Total	790	100.0	189	100.0	979	100.0
Ethnicity						
White	466	59.0	173	91.5	639	65.3
Black	281	35.6	11	5.8	292	29.8
Hispanic	30	3.8	3	1.6	33	3.4
Other	6	0.8	0	0.0	6	0.6
No answer	7	0.9	2	1.0	9	0.9
Total	790	100.1	189	99.9	979	100.0

TABLE **C-1** *Continued*

Characteristic	Urban		Nonurban		Total	
	No.	Percent	No.	Percent	No.	Percent
Age (years)						
18–29	250	31.6	90	47.6	340	34.7
30–39	224	28.4	46	24.3	270	27.6
40–49	139	17.6	25	13.2	164	16.8
50–59	115	14.6	15	7.9	130	13.3
⩾60	53	6.7	10	5.3	63	6.4
No answer	9	1.1	3	1.6	12	1.2
Total	790	100.0	139	99.9	979	100.0
Education						
No formal schooling	7	0.9	1	0.5	8	0.8
1–8 grades	129	16.3	32	16.9	161	16.4
9–11 grades	291	36.8	73	38.6	364	37.2
High school graduate	241	30.5	57	30.2	298	30.4
Some college	97	12.3	22	11.6	119	12.2
College graduate	19	2.4	3	1.6	22	2.3
No answer	6	0.8	1	0.5	7	0.7
Total	790	100.0	199	99.9	979	100.0
Marital Status						
Married	53	6.7	35	18.5	88	9.0
Separated	114	14.4	21	11.1	135	13.8
Widowed	39	4.9	4	2.1	43	4.4
Divorced	199	25.2	48	25.4	247	25.2
Never been married	366	46.3	72	38.1	438	44.7
Living together	12	1.5	9	4.8	21	2.1
No answer	7	0.9	0	0.0	7	0.7
Total	790	99.9	189	100.0	979	99.9
Veteran status						
Yes	264	33.4	46	24.3	310	31.7
(Vietnam veteran)	(73)	(9.2)	(10)	(5.3)	(83)	(8.5)
No	523	66.2	142	75.1	665	67.9
No answer	3	0.4	1	0.5	4	0.4
Total	790	100.0	189	99.9	979	100.0
Ever been in jail/prison						
Yes	470	59.5	103	54.5	573	58.5
No	313	39.5	85	45.0	398	40.7
No answer	7	0.9	1	0.5	8	0.8
Total	790	100.0	189	100.0	979	100.0

SOURCE: Ohio Department of Mental Health (1985).

(Vermont Department of Human Services, 1985). They also reflect the profile of farmers who have recently lost their land: they are young and well-educated (Brown and Deavers, no date). There are no appreciable differences between urban and rural homeless on education or incarceration.

Military Service

The urban homeless are more likely to have served in the military (33.4 percent) than are their rural counterparts (24.3 percent).

Homelessness

Nearly three-quarters of both the urban and rural respondents had been homeless for less than 1 year (Table C-2). A slightly higher percentage of urban respondents had been homeless for more than 2 years.

Reason for Homelessness

When asked to identify the major cause of their homelessness, both groups overwhelmingly cited economic factors as the most important reason and family problems as the second most important (Table C-3). These responses parallel the available anecdotal and descriptive data from other studies.

TABLE C-2   Length of Time Respondents Were Homeless (Ohio Data)

Time (days)	Urban		Nonurban		Total	
	No.	Percent	No.	Percent	No.	Percent
≤30	308	39.0	73	38.6	381	38.9
31–60	71	9.0	25	13.2	96	9.8
61–365	192	24.3	46	24.3	238	24.3
366–730	50	6.3	17	9.0	67	6.8
≥731	126	16.0	21	11.1	147	15.0
No answer	43	5.4	7	3.7	50	5.1
Total	790	100.0	189	99.9	979	99.9
Mean no. of days	675.9		378.4		617.6	
Median no. of days	60.0		60.0		60.0	

SOURCE: Ohio Department of Mental Health (1985).

TABLE C-3   Reported Major Reason for Homelessness (Ohio Data)

Reason	Urban No.	Urban Percent	Nonurban No.	Nonurban Percent	Total No.	Total Percent
Unemployment	173	21.9	40	21.2	213	21.7
Problems paying rent	111	14.1	25	13.2	136	13.9
Family conflict	100	12.7	30	15.9	130	13.3
Eviction	74	9.4	20	10.6	94	9.6
Other reasons	70	8.9	22	11.6	92	9.4
Family dissolution	54	6.8	24	12.7	78	8.0
Alcohol/drug abuse	63	8.0	8	4.2	71	7.3
Like to move around	52	6.6	8	4.2	60	6.1
Government benefits stopped	27	3.4	0	0.0	27	2.8
Disaster	20	2.5	4	2.1	24	2.5
Deinstitutionalization	18	2.3	6	3.2	24	2.5
Was in jail/prison	15	1.9	1	0.5	16	1.6
No answer	13	1.5	1	0.5	14	1.4
Total	790	100.1	199	99.9	979	100.1

SOURCE: Ohio Department of Mental Health (1985).

Shelter

The rural homeless are four times more likely to have spent the previous night with family or friends (40.7 versus 10.7 percent for urban homeless), while the urban homeless are far more likely to rely on missions or shelters for lodging (37.1 versus 11.1 percent) (Table C-4). This is one case in which it is helpful to disaggregate the data to look at the use of shelters by the nonurban homeless. As expected, the data confirm that these shelters are most likely located in the urbanized (or mixed) rural communities. In fact, only 20.4 percent of the homeless in these urbanized rural communities used shelters or missions, while none of those in more rural counties had spent a night in these facilities.

Transience

Both the urban and rural homeless do not move as often as one might expect (Table C-5); in fact, over half of both groups spent the previous month in only one or two lodgings.

In Table C-6, there is a striking but not unexpected contrast in the reasons for which the urban and rural homeless moved to the county in which they were interviewed. While 22 percent of the urban homeless

TABLE C-4   Place Respondents Slept the Previous Night (Ohio Data)

Place	Urban		Nonurban		Total	
	No.	Percent	No.	Percent	No.	Percent
Limited or no shelter	238	30.1	50	26.5	288	29.4
No shelter	131	16.6	30	15.9	161	16.4
Car, abandoned building, public facility	107	13.5	20	10.6	127	13.0
Mission, shelter	293	37.1	21	11.1	314	32.1
Cheap motels and hotels	141	17.8	30	15.9	171	17.5
Other	116	14.7	88	46.6	204	20.8
With family	28	3.5	32	16.9	60	6.1
With friends	57	7.2	45	23.8	102	10.4
Unique conditions	31	3.9	11	5.8	42	4.3
No answer	2	0.2	0	0.0	2	0.2
Total	790	99.9	189	100.1	979	100.0

SOURCE: Ohio Department of Mental Health (1985).

came in search of a job, only 8 percent of the rural homeless did so. For the rural homeless, the overwhelming reason (43.7 percent) was to be near friends and relatives (only 19.7 percent of urban homeless gave that response).

Employment

Based on self-reports by nonurban homeless individuals, the findings on employment suggest that they had a more recent attachment to the

TABLE C-5   Number of Places the Homeless Stayed During the Previous Month (Ohio Data)

No. of Places	Urban		Nonurban		Total	
	No.	Percent	No.	Percent	No.	Percent
1–2	453	57.3	106	56.1	559	57.1
3–4	188	23.8	57	30.2	245	25.0
5–6	55	7.0	14	7.4	69	7.0
7–8	17	2.2	3	1.6	20	2.0
>8	50	6.3	7	3.7	57	5.8
No answer	27	3.4	2	1.1	29	3.0
Total	790	100.0	189	100.1	979	99.9
Mean number	3.3		3.1		3.3	
Median number	2.0		2.0		2.0	

SOURCE: Ohio Department of Mental Health (1985).

TABLE C-6   Reason for Nonpermanent Residents Coming to County (Ohio Data)

	Urban		Nonurban		Total	
Reason	No.	Percent	No.	Percent	No.	Percent
To live with relative or friend	90	19.7	59	43.7	149	25.1
To look for a job	101	22.1	11	8.1	112	19.0
Other reasons	63	13.8	24	17.8	87	14.7
Another stop while passing through	48	10.5	13	9.6	61	10.3
To take a job	40	8.8	12	8.9	52	8.8
For public sleeping shelters	30	6.6	3	2.2	33	5.6
Lived here before	25	5.5	9	6.7	34	5.8
For social service programs	8	1.8	1	0.7	9	1.5
To go to school	9	2.0	0	0.0	9	1.5
Heard you could get on welfare	4	0.9	2	1.5	6	1.0
For community kitchens	4	0.9	0	0.0	4	0.7
Less police hassle	2	0.3	0	0.0	2	0.4
No answer	32	7.0	1	0.7	33	5.5
Total	456	100.0	135	99.9	591	100.0

SOURCE: Ohio Department of Mental Health (1985).

labor force and current earnings were a much more important source of revenue for those with any income. Some of the data are summarized below:

- Ever held a job (percentage who held a job at some point)?
—Urban homeless: 85.9
—Nonurban homeless: 93.6

- Worked in the last month (percentage who reported working)?
—Urban homeless: 22.2
—Nonurban homeless: 35.4
    Mixed county: 42.7
    Rural county: 25.7

- The last year worked for those who have not worked in the previous month (percentage).
—Urban homeless   —Nonurban homeless
   1983–1984:   33.6   1983–1984:   54.5
   1978–1982:   38.6   1978–1982:   30.0

- Reason for not working now.

Two major reasons (percentage)	Urban Homeless	Nonurban Homeless
Looked, but cannot find work:	43.9	61.8
Disabled; cannot find work:	21.7	16.4

COUNTING THE HOMELESS

There are no reliable estimates of the number of rural homeless. Few states have even published estimates of the number of rural homeless clients that are served by social service providers. Two that did, California (California Department of Economic Opportunity, 1986) and Maryland, (Maryland Department of Human Resources, 1986) developed identical estimates: 18 percent of the homeless are rural residents.* Despite the striking similarities of the data from these two states, it would be premature to attempt national estimates at this point based on these figures. Service provider estimates are often biased upward as a result of counting the same individual or family twice when they are served by the same provider at different times or by multiple providers. At the same time, it is clear that many aspects of the rural environment contribute to the invisibility of the rural homeless, leading to the potential for underestimates.

First, the problems of enumerating the homeless in the urban area multiply in the vast geographic expanse of rural America. As noted earlier, service providers are seldom found outside the larger rural communities (Redburn and Buss, 1987); therefore, provider-based surveys only tap a portion of the homeless in rural communities. In addition, there are difficult methodological problems in counting those homeless people who are temporarily sheltered with friends, neighbors, and relatives, an issue requiring further empirical work. In addition, as the Ohio study demonstrated, there are difficulties in identifying those rural homeless who are outside of rural communities:

. . . hermits who live in caves, culverts or lean-tos; mountain people who have had a bad year in a kind of hunting/gathering society; miners who have been laid off; homeless persons who prefer the woods to the streets; and others who have exiled themselves. These homeless people are, in many ways, indistinguishable from mountain or rural people who are poor but not homeless.

Nearly all of these people, the homeless and others alike, appear to have two things in common: they are heavily armed; and they do not like strangers. (Redburn and Buss, 1987)

Second, there is a major perceptual issue regarding the concept of homelessness. The very nature of the informal support system in rural areas leads residents to view homelessness as an attribute of transients and outsiders. Community residents who have lost their farms or homes are constantly referred to as "local folks on hard times," while outsiders or transients are more readily labeled as homeless. To the extent that the local community serves few transients or outsiders, residents generally

---

*The Ohio data presented here cannot be used to project the number of rural homeless in the state. The rural homeless were oversampled.

do not perceive the fact that homelessness exists in their community. Thus, even surveys that go beyond social service providers to key community leaders can still result in underestimates.

All of these factors converge to make rural homelessness, like rural poverty, difficult to assess and measure. From a public policy perspective, the central question may not be the actual number of rural homeless but the ability of local communities to meet that burden without outside assistance from the federal or state government.

THE RURAL ENVIRONMENT

To understand the ability of rural communities to respond to the growing number of homeless people, it is important to consider aspects of the rural environment that affect both the capability and inclination of rural communities to respond.

The starting point for any discussion of rural America is an examination of the diversity of rural communities; the importance of this diversity cannot be overemphasized. Rural Arizona is a very different place from rural Alabama or rural Minnesota. These differences are far from trivial.

In fact, the National Rural Health Association has identified at least four types of rural communities:

• Adjacent rural areas—contiguous to or within metropolitan statistical areas (MSAs), which are very similar to their urban neighbors;

• Urbanized rural areas—population of 25,000 or more but distant from an MSA;

• Frontier areas—population densities of less than 6 people per square mile; these are the most remote areas; there are no frontier areas east of the Mississippi River; and

• Countryside rural areas—the remainder of the country not covered by urban or rural designations. (Elison, no date)

Both community size and proximity to urban areas have a profound impact on a community's ability to develop and maintain a formal social services network for its residents and the homeless in its midst.

Larger Rural Communities

The larger rural communities generally have a broader economic base and a more formalized social services network (Ohio Department of Mental Health, 1985); the bulk of rural shelters and community kitchens appear to be located in these communities (Redburn and Buss, 1987). While many of the poorer or more remote rural communities face serious obstacles in attracting sufficient numbers of health care providers, there is less of a problem in larger communities. During the site visits to these communities, the committee found shelters that generally had direct access to health care professionals or that encouraged their residents to secure health care, through federal programs or Medicaid or other state programs, as quickly as possible.

A number of observations regarding these communities can be made as a result of the site visits. First, demand for overnight and emergency shelters clearly outstripped the supply, as did requests to the local food pantries. Many shelters were operating at capacity; in fact, one shelter was licensed for 10 residents but was housing 25 residents at the time of the site visit. Community Action Agency staff often reported that their annual budget for the provision of emergency housing services was depleted in the first 2 to 3 months of the fiscal year. Similarly, social service organizations often found that their monthly funds for housing vouchers were exhausted early in the month.

Second, there were few facilities that could accommodate an intact family, and fewer still that could accept underage youths.

Third, despite the obvious distress in the local farm economy, few displaced farmers or farmhands made use of these shelters. Future research needs to focus on what happens to these farmers and farmhands following foreclosure and what support services, if any, they actually utilize.

Finally, shelter staff, homeless advocates, and the social service community were quite innovative in their approach to problems. A few examples follow.

• Tired of finding chronically mentally ill patients on his doorstep without warning, the director of one center has succeeded in enlisting the cooperation of one of the state mental hospitals in an effort to work together to plan for a patient's discharge. He is now trying to elicit the cooperation of the other major state mental hospital.

• In an effort to develop a more effective long-term intervention strategy, the development of transitional housing was moving ahead with surprising speed in Minnesota. Transitional housing provides a more permanent living environment (generally up to 6 months) for those homeless individuals capable of living independently, facilitating job search and reentry into the community.

• The Dorothy Day House in Minnesota also has begun operation of a farm in an effort to develop a place where the "burnt out" homeless, consumed by the daily struggle for survival, could have several months in a peaceful, remote setting to renew themselves.

• An innovative peer counseling program was developed for farmers

by a Catholic Charities family service agency in an effort to brea
self-imposed isolation of troubled farm families. To encourage p
pation, they ensured anonymity for farmers seeking counseling by drawing
their counselors from farm families on the other side of the county. A
secondary aim of the program was to provide financial assistance to the
farmers and counselors, who were well reimbursed for their time.

Smaller Rural Communities

Smaller rural communities seldom have a formal social services system.
Instead, they have a highly developed informal referral network among
the leading members of the community that can be mobilized to assist
community residents in need. Transients requiring assistance present an
entirely different situation; they are often given short shrift. They are
highly visible strangers and are generally viewed with suspicion. As the
Ohio researchers discovered, rural leaders

. . . perceive their systems to be targeted almost exclusively to local homeless
residents as opposed to transients or outsiders. Transients or outsiders are usually
encouraged, often by force, to move on to urban areas. This is accomplished by
providing bus fare to the nearest city, arresting persons until deportation can be
executed, "rousting" persons from public and private places, and offering or
providing few, if any, helping services. Non-urban places are hostile to homeless
outsiders. (Ohio Department of Mental Health, 1985)

Yet there are growing indications, found both during the site visits and
in the literature, that these communities are not always mobilizing to
support neighbors in financial distress as they have in the past. This was
most evident in the farming communities. Farmers have always been an
independent group, and usually are quite unwilling to ask for assistance.
In the past, such a request never had to be made: neighbors simply
showed up to help. That spirit of rural cooperation is best typified by the
traditional barn raising.

While farmers still believe that their neighbors will assist them in the
event of death or natural catastrophe, the farmers who had recently faced
foreclosure did so alone. During the site visit to Minnesota, farmers
spoke bitterly of the decline of the old rural ethic that "we take care of
our own." Their stories echoed a recent *Wall Street Journal* article, in
which troubled farm families claimed that they were "shunned in church,
taunted in schools and often subsisting on skimpy meals" (Wall, 1985).

Farmers attributed this change in attitude to a number of factors. Over
the last two decades changing farm technology has eliminated the need
for collective efforts such as group harvesting. Farms have become more

insulated from each other; they are becoming more of a business than a neighborly family operation. There is a new prevailing attitude; if a neighbor is in trouble, it must be his or her own fault for becoming financially overextended. Perhaps more important, the farm crisis is so pervasive that many neighbors are barely able to maintain subsistence and have little to share. A study of 40 families forced out of farming in Missouri confirms impressions from the Minnesota site visit that there is a "surprising lack of support reportedly provided these families by their communities" (Heffernan and Heffernan, 1986). The fraying of the social support fabric in these rural communities could have important implications for the rate at which financially troubled families descend into homelessness.

Farm families also singled out the food stamp program as an example of the failure of publicly funded income support programs to prevent this downward spiral. They were convinced that timely assistance from existing programs could have prevented many farm families from entering the ranks of the homeless, and were particularly bitter at the failure of public officials to recognize how the eligibility criteria for these programs systematically disqualified farm families.

Inadequate Housing

The U.S. Department of Housing and Urban Development has estimated that in 1983, 840,000 members of very-low-income rural households were living in "severely inadequate" housing; members of another million very-low-income households were living in houses that were merely "inadequate" (Wilson, 1983).*

Adequate affordable housing was a major issue in all of the states that the committee visited. While there was an extensive series of subsidized and public housing projects in the rural towns in the South, they were not sufficient to meet the demand, and waiting lists often stretched for years. As a result, many local residents were forced to live in extremely substandard dwellings, essentially, broken-down shacks, for which most paid a rent of $25 per month. A few had indoor plumbing; most did not. A few more had an outdoor privy; at least half of these shacks lacked even a privy.

In Minnesota, substandard, low-cost housing of the type seen in southern states could not be found. Displaced farmers and rural workers faced a different dilemma: rental rates two to three times the level they had paid in their smaller communities.

---

*The U.S. Department of Housing and Urban Development defines very-low-income households as those with incomes below 50 percent of the area median.

Transportation

Transportation remains one of the greatest barriers to access for rural health and social services as well as employment opportunities. The problem can be measured both in distance and travel time. It is further complicated by unpredictable weather, which can make travel both risky and inefficient.

While states such as Alabama have a strong outreach program through their child protective service and public health nurse program, access to physician services, even when free, is often thwarted by transportation barriers. During the Alabama site visit, many of the rural poor noted that their neighbors charged them $10 to $20 for a ride to the local health clinic. That nearly equalled a month's rent for many of these families and made such trips prohibitively expensive, unless there was a true emergency.

Homeless people served by some community health care centers, such as the one in Mound Bayou, Mississippi, are more fortunate. The health care center is able to provide bus service throughout the rural counties. Once again, however, the cost in time to those being served appears high. The bus follows a fixed route, meaning that for some clinic users, a routine visit consumes an entire day: a several-mile walk to and from the bus stop; a bus ride that might take as long as 2 hours each way, and the time at the clinic.

Transportation barriers also discourage participation in vital nutrition assistance programs such as food stamps. A recent report by the Food Research and Action Council noted that:

A total of 40 Texas counties, more than 15% of those in the state, do not have a food stamp office. . . . [C]onsequently, some persons may have to travel upwards of 50 miles to apply for public assistance benefits.

Clients receiving $10 to $15 in food stamps sometimes have to pay that much to get to the office.

(Or in Arkansas): Many persons have to pay someone to drive them [on] a 100 mile round trip only to be refused to be seen if they are 15 minutes late. (Food Research and Action Council, 1987)

HEALTH CARE RESOURCES

In the last three decades, a number of federal initiatives were designed to increase the accessibility of health care in rural areas: the national Hill-Burton Hospital Construction Program, the establishment of community mental health centers and community and migrant health centers in underserved areas, and the development of the National Health Service Corps. While access to care has clearly improved for many rural residents, it remains problematic for many others.

There are a number of barriers to access that remain, the most prominent of which is financial. The majority of rural poor live in intact families, but the states in which they live generally do not extend Medicaid eligibility to intact two-parent families and set eligibility levels for single mothers at a fraction of the federal poverty level. Because of the preponderance of minimum wage jobs in the service sector that have few benefits, the working poor are also less likely to be insured. Insurance is often unaffordable: Premiums on individual policies are high and must be paid without the benefit of either a contribution by the employer or the tax subsidy of employment-based insurance.

Even when families have health insurance, financial barriers may remain. A recent survey of financially distressed rural Minnesota farm families indicated that while most farm families struggled to retain their health insurance coverage as their economic situation deteriorated, they had been forced to maintain a high deductible rate and curtail their use of discretionary preventive care, such as mammograms or Pap smears (Southern Minnesota Family Farm Fund, 1986).

As a result, unforeseen emergency care may have the double impact of providing the financial push from poverty to homelessness for rural residents, depleting the family's remaining resources, and, at the same time, effectively divorcing the family from future access to care. The adequacy of Medicaid coverage for the poor and near poor is a major issue in preventing homelessness and ensuring continuing care should homelessness occur for other reasons.

Another barrier is limited provider availability. Rural areas attract fewer health care providers: Salaries are lower, as are third-party insurance reimbursement levels; there are fewer professional support systems or health care facilities; and, there is less potential for continuing education. David Kindig of the University of Wisconsin recently reported that the level of physician availability for counties with populations of less than 10,000 is one-third the national average, the growth of physician availability in rural areas over the last decade (14.2 percent) was significantly less than that in the nation as a whole (32.5 percent), and in general, smaller counties have lower physician availability (Kindig and Movassaghi, 1987).

Other traditional sources of care are in transition. Rural hospitals have faced more significant declines in admissions, patient length of stay, and occupancy rates than their urban counterparts, while they have experienced reimbursement constraints from Medicare and other insurers (Congressional Research Service, 1986). The results have been an increase in the number of closures of rural hospitals and a declining financial situation for many rural hospitals, severely limiting their ability to provide uncompensated care.

The resources of community health centers, the primary source of health care for many of the rural poor, have been limited by declining federal resources throughout the economic recession of the 1980s. With increased need and fewer dollars, community health centers have been prodded by federal officials to expand both the number of private pay patients they see and the amount of private pay collections in an effort to broaden their resource base. While marketing to paying clients was intended to bring in the necessary revenue to continue outreach services to the underserved and to subsidize services to the centers' poorer clients, such efforts have not always been successful. In addition, in areas such as dental care, budget constraints appear to be replacing curative work with lower cost prevention efforts.

At the same time that access to health resources is constrained, the rural poor and homeless often appear to face greater health risks. As the site visit to Alabama's Black Belt demonstrated, rural poverty itself can pose a grave environmental threat to health. Substandard housing lacking insulation or even a privy increases the risk of contaminated water supplies, the spread of infectious diseases, and accidents. In such an environment, it is often impossible to maintain proper nutrition; storage and preparation of foods are hindered by the conditions of these shacks and of the major appliances; and early childhood development is retarded by the lack of intellectual stimulation and the inability to develop a sense of self-esteem. As in the urban ghetto, the limited funds available to these families to purchase a balanced diet are eroded even further by an inability to travel to grocery stores that have lower prices.

Health Care for the Homeless

The U.S. Department of Health and Human Services (HHS), in support of this appendix, recently asked its 10 regional offices to survey their community and migrant health center grantees serving rural populations to determine the utilization of health services by the homeless. While all of the regional reports are not yet available, the report from the Chicago Region V office (covering Illinois, Indiana, Michigan, Minnesota, Ohio, and Wisconsin) provides the most comprehensive data of those now available (C. Tavani, personal communication).

These results must be viewed with some caution. The survey was not scientific. In responding to this survey, centers did not conduct a comprehensive review of their caseload in an attempt to identify the homeless and their health care problems. Thus, the possibility of under-counting the homeless is high. Community health centers do not regularly attempt to identify whether patients are homeless. In fact, most patients generally provide the centers' staff with an address when asked, even if they provide an out-of-date or fictional address or the address of a friend or relative.

Of the 36 community and migrant health centers surveyed in the Midwest, 29 reported that they had served homeless patients (Table C-7) during the previous year. With a range from 4 to 120 patients per year, the median annual number of homeless patients served was 25.

The major health problems of the rural homeless are identified in Table C-8. Acute and episodic illnesses (including colds, upper respiratory disturbances, gastrointestinal disturbances, and dermatological problems) and malnutrition lead the list. Reports from other regional offices (not presented here) suggest the importance of substance abuse and mental health needs; these problems were highlighted during the site visits. The use of alternative service providers, such as detoxification centers, may be an important factor in the lower frequency of substance abuse reported here. Regarding mental health services, even in the larger rural communities, access to mental health professionals is limited for indigent populations. The extremely large catchment areas for community mental health centers and the limited resources for treating a diverse rural population pose severe access barriers.

The site visits also highlighted a tremendous need for curative dental services among the rural homeless and poor. In most cases, preventive care was of little value to these individuals. To the extent that community health centers have been forced by budget constraints to emphasize preventive care over curative dental services, the frequency reflected in Table C-8 may be artificially low.

Table C-9 highlights the type of services received by the rural homeless. In addition to primary care, additional services were provided to the homeless either on site or by referral. The social services category includes temporary shelter, clothing, food, emergency welfare, the special

TABLE C-7   Estimated Number of Homeless Served by Health Center (Chicago HHS Region V Data)

	Ill.	Ind.	Mich.	Minn.	Ohio	Wis.	Total
Median	28	100	25	63	31	6	25
Range							
Low	4		5	25	12	4	4
High	47		50	100	120	40	120
No. of centers	6	1	11	2	6	3	29

SOURCE: C. Tavani, Office of Planning, Evaluation, and Legislation, Health Resources and Services Administration, U.S. Department of Health and Human Services, Washington, D.C. Personal communication.

TABLE C-8   Major Health Problems of the Rural Homeless (Chicago HHS Region V Data)

Problem	Frequency in:						
	Ill.	Ind.	Mich.	Minn.	Ohio	Wis.	Total
Acute/episodic illness[a]	6	1	9	1	3	2	22
Malnutrition	5	1	9	2	4	1	22
Alcoholism/drug abuse	1	1	3	1	3	1	10
Emergency	2		4	1	2	1	10
Dental	2		4		1	1	8
Mental health	1	1	2	1	2		7
Chronic illness[b]	1		3	1	1		6
Hypothermia/overexposure	1	1	1	1	1		5
Maternity/obstetrics/gynecology	2		2		1		5
Hygiene/sanitation	1		2				3
Seek pain medication			1			1	2
Other[c]			2		1		3

[a]Includes upper respiratory, gastrointestinal, dermatological, and similar disturbances.
[b]Includes diabetes, cardiovascular, hypertensive, arthritic, and similar disturbances.
[c]Includes general malaise, neglected medical attention, and similar conditions.

SOURCE: C. Tavani, Office of Planning, Evaluation, and Legislation, Health Resources and Services Administration, U.S. Department of Health and Human Services, Washington, D.C. Personal communication.

supplemental food program for Women, Infants, and Children (WIC), and similar services. The frequency of nutritional counseling attests to the importance of nutrition as a health risk factor in this population.

THE OHIO MENTAL HEALTH STUDY

Unfortunately, the data presented above do not permit a comparison with the urban homeless population; for such a comparison, the only source of statistical data, once again, is the Ohio Mental Health Study.

Health Status

The Ohio Mental Health Study asked the homeless to identify their physical health problems; the answers are presented in Table C-10. Overall, 30.7 percent of respondents reported a current medical problem; no striking differences emerged from the data for the urban and nonurban homeless. The differences between this list and the one presented by the Chicago Region V office in Table C-8 may reflect reporting bias; these

TABLE C-9 Services Provided to Rural Homeless (Chicago HHS Region V Data)

Type of Service	Frequency of Response						
	Ill.	Ind.	Mich.	Minn.	Ohio	Wis.	Total
Primary care	5	1	11	2	6	2	27
Social services	3	1	6	1	5	2	18
Nutrition	5	1	5	1	2		14
Dental	1		4	1	1		7
Health education	1		1	2	2		6
Transportation	1		2	1	2		6
Pharmacy	2		2	1	1		6
Specialized medical care	1		1		1	1	4
Mental health		1	2		1		4
Translation	1			1		1	3
Substance abuse						1	1

SOURCE: C. Tavani, Office of Planning, Evaluation, and Legislation, Health Resources and Services Administration, U.S. Department of Health and Human Services, Washington, D.C. Personal communication.

data are based on self-reports; the Midwest data are based on provider recall. There were no data available on the rural homeless based on chart review or actual patient exams. The limitations of self-reporting are best demonstrated by the limited recognition by the rural homeless that they face dental problems. Health care providers and the site visits substantiated that dental problems are among the most significant of the unmet health care needs of the rural homeless.

An interesting finding resulted when the data for the nonurban group were disaggregated into a rural county category and a mixed (urbanized rural) county category. Significant differences emerged in the overall rate of reported illness: In comparison with 31 percent of the urban homeless who reported a health problem, the mixed (urbanized rural) county rate was 20.4 percent while the rate for rural homeless was 41 percent. Unfortunately, a table disaggregating the specific health problems was not available. One possible explanation for the higher rural rate would be the very high accident rate in farming that might leave former farm laborers with residual chronic problems.

Emergency Room Utilization

The overall rate of emergency room utilization by the homeless was only slightly higher than that for the general population (Table C-11). In

1984 Redburn and Buss (1987) reported that 23 percent of the adult population in Ohio reported that they had been to an emergency room in the previous year, compared with 25 percent of the homeless overall.

Table C-11 shows that the nonurban homeless use emergency rooms at a slightly higher rate (29.6 percent); the urban homeless use emergency rooms at a level closer to that for the general population (23 percent).

Despite the lack of alternative primary care providers, the voluntary use of emergency rooms may actually be far lower than these numbers suggest. Very often emergency room visits are instigated by local

TABLE **C-10**   Physical Health Problems Identified by Homeless People (Ohio Data)

	Urban		Nonurban		Total	
Problem	No.	Percent	No.	Percent	No.	Percent
Reported no physical problems	536	67.8	133	70.4	669	68.3
Reported physical problems	245	31.0	56	29.6	301	30.7
Ill-defined conditions	70	8.9	19	10.0	89	9.1
Arthritis, rheumatism, and other diseases of the musculoskeletal system	38	4.8	11	5.8	49	5.0
Injury and poisoning	38	4.8	4	2.1	42	4.3
Diseases of the heart and circulatory system	33	4.2	5	2.6	38	3.9
Diseases of the nervous system and sense organs	27	3.4	7	3.7	34	3.5
Diseases of the respiratory system	24	3.0	6	3.2	30	3.1
Diseases of the digestive system	21	2.7	7	3.7	28	2.9
Eye problems	18	2.3	4	2.1	22	2.2
Endocrine and nutritional disorders	14	1.8	4	2.1	18	1.8
Dental problems	14	1.8	2	1.0	16	1.6
Infections and parasitic disorders	8	1.0	3	1.6	11	1.1
Neoplasms (cancer and benign tumors)	7	0.9	3	1.6	10	1.0
Diseases of the genitourinary system	6	0.7	4	2.1	10	1.0
Pregnancy	6	0.7	3	1.6	9	0.9
Diseases of the blood	6	0.7	2	1.0	8	0.8
Alcoholism	6	0.7	0	0.0	6	0.6
Diseases of the skin	4	0.5	0	0.0	4	0.4
No answer	2	0.2	2	1.0	4	0.4
No answer	9	1.1	0	0.0	9	0.9
Total	790	100.0	189	100.0	979	99.9

NOTE: Subtotals for types of problems do not add to the values for "Reported physical problems" because 127 respondents indicated they had two problems.

SOURCE: Ohio Department of Mental Health (1985).

TABLE C-11   Social Service Usage by Homeless People (Ohio Data)

Social Service	Urban		Nonurban		Total	
	No.	Percent	No.	Percent	No.	Percent
Community kitchens	531	67.2	64	33.8	595	60.8
Shelters	506	64.0	46	24.3	552	56.4
Welfare/general relief	319	40.4	116	61.4	435	44.4
Hospital emergency rooms	184	23.3	56	29.6	240	24.5
Shelters for battered women	21	18.6	2	4.0	23	12.4
Community mental health centers	91	11.5	28	14.8	119	12.2

SOURCE: Ohio Department of Mental Health (1985).

authorities if a homeless person is arrested for drunkenness, substance abuse, or loss of emotional control (Redburn and Buss, 1987). The decision to take the person to the emergency room is often a pragmatic move in an effort to limit the potential liability of the authorities in these cases if anything should go wrong.

More often than not, the homeless only use the health care system at times of mental or physical health crisis.

Psychiatric Hospitalization

The number of homeless people in Ohio that have been deinstitution-alized does not reflect the previous high estimates of the deinstitutionalized identified in earlier studies. For both the urban and rural homeless, 3 out of 10 were hospitalized for emotional or mental health problems at some point in their lives (Table C-12).

The Ohio study concluded that the urban homeless "exhibit rates of psychiatric symptoms similar to the rural homeless but show higher rates of behavioral disturbance" (Redburn and Buss, 1987).

Alcohol Abuse

As much as one-third of the total homeless population has problems with alcohol or drugs. The available data (Tables C-13 and C-14) suggest that alcoholism poses a larger problem for the urban homeless. Twice as many urban homeless reported that they drank a lot during the previous month (21.3 percent for the urban homeless versus 10.6 percent for the nonurban homeless). In addition, nearly 3 out of 10 urban homeless reported that they had sought help for their alcoholism, compared with 20.1 percent of the nonurban homeless population.

TABLE C-12   Psychiatric Hospitalization Reported by Homeless People (Ohio Data)

Hospitalization	Urban		Nonurban		Total	
	No.	Percent	No.	Percent	No.	Percent
Never been hospitalized	536	67.8	137	72.5	673	68.7
Been hospitalized[a]	242	30.6	51	27.0	293	29.9
Veteran's hospital	55	7.0	5	2.6	60	6.1
General hospital	100	12.7	29	15.3	129	13.2
State hospital	155	19.6	25	13.2	180	18.4
No answer	12	1.5	1	0.5	13	1.3
Total	790	99.9	189	100.0	979	99.9

[a]Hospitalized subtotals do not add to the percentages listed as "Been hospitalized" because some respondents had hospitalizations in more than one type of setting.

SOURCE: Ohio Department of Mental Health (1985).

TABLE C-13   Reported Drinking by Homeless People During the Previous Month (Ohio Data)

Amount of Drinking	Urban		Nonurban		Total	
	No.	Percent	No.	Percent	No.	Percent
Some	349	44.2	92	48.7	441	45.0
A lot	168	21.3	20	10.6	188	19.2
Not at all	268	33.9	77	40.7	345	35.2
No answer	5	0.6	0	0.0	5	0.5
Total	790	100.0	189	100.0	979	99.9

NOTE: Urban (28.1 percent) homeless people were somewhat more likely to report seeking help for a drinking problem than were nonurban people (20.1 percent). This may be the result of service availability in urban versus nonurban areas.

SOURCE: Ohio Department of Mental Health (1985).

TABLE C-14   Reported Seeking Help for Drinking by Homeless People (Ohio Data)

Behavior	No.	Percent of Total
Have ever sought help	260	26.6
Have not sought help	693	70.8
No answer	26	2.7
Total	979	100.1

SOURCE: Ohio Department of Mental Health (1985).

General Well-Being

Tables C-15 and C-16 suggest that the homeless population has a far more optimistic self-evaluation than might be expected. A large percentage rate their outlook positively, and nearly a third of both groups described their lives as satisfying. There are no significant differences between the two groups on these measures.

Overall, the available data and the site visits suggest that the health care needs of the rural homeless are not significantly different from those of their urban counterparts. It is important to reemphasize, however, that the existing data base is quite meager.

The major health care problems among the adult population are malnutrition, alcoholism and substance abuse, dental care, respiratory illness, stress, depression, mental illness, and environmental health problems such as those related to impure drinking water.

While there is little continuity of care, access to acute health care services seems adequate if there is a pressing physical health problem. Routine or preventive care services are seldom sought because of significant barriers to access, shame, or hostility toward the health care system.

Access to mental health professionals is different, however. Not only are services limited but there is every indication that there is an unmet need for such services among the chronically mentally ill and specific homeless groups, such as farmers. The chronically mentally ill often have trouble accessing the available resources; in general, farmers will not or cannot utilize the available resources because of strong conservative cultural forces (McCormick, 1987). Among teenagers, venereal disease and pregnancy are the two major health issues; little prenatal care is

TABLE C-15   Self-Ratings by Homeless People of Their Nerves, Spirits, Outlook, or Mental Health at Present (Ohio Data)

Response	Urban		Nonurban		Total	
	No.	Percent	No.	Percent	No.	Percent
Excellent	77	9.7	13	6.9	90	9.2
Good	239	30.2	66	34.9	305	31.2
Fair	274	34.7	64	33.9	338	34.5
Poor	125	15.8	27	14.3	152	15.5
Very bad	60	7.6	17	9.0	77	7.9
No answer	15	1.9	2	1.1	17	1.7
Total	790	99.9	189	100.1	979	99.9

SOURCE: Ohio Department of Mental Health (1985).

TABLE C-16 Self-Ratings by Homeless People of Their Satisfaction with Life (Ohio Data)

Response	Urban		Nonurban		Total	
	No.	Percent	No.	Percent	No.	Percent
Very satisfying	80	10.1	16	8.5	96	9.8
Somewhat satisfying	189	23.9	43	22.7	232	23.7
Mixed	282	35.7	78	41.3	360	36.8
Not very satisfying	161	20.4	35	18.5	196	20.0
Not at all satisfying	63	8.0	16	8.5	79	8.1
No answer	15	1.9	1	0.5	16	1.6
Total	790	100.0	189	100.0	979	100.0

SOURCE: Ohio Department of Mental Health (1985).

provided in the South until the final trimester. As in other areas, the malpractice crisis has limited the number of physicians willing to handle obstetrical cases.

Children suffer from malnutrition and failure to thrive, and are at serious risk of accidents, particularly those living in substandard dwellings. They also fail to receive the necessary preventive care. The consequences of this can be devastating.

The depression, stress, and suicidal tendencies among the farm population warrant special outreach efforts in the view of most of our key informants. They strongly suggest that suicides in the farm community are deliberately misreported by the families to save face, that spouse and child abuse rates are rising in this population group, and that alcoholism is increasing. Senator David Durenberger's report of trends in services in southwestern Minnesota may be indicative: according to the senator, a mental health worker in that region stated that between 1983 and 1985 her center experienced a 330 percent increase in the number of people using the 24-hour crisis line and a 30 percent increase in the number of outpatient mental health services (U.S. Congress, Senate, Committee on Finance, 1986).

Teenagers who live on farms appear to be having a particularly rough time. In some cases, their entire lives are preordained: First, they become members of 4-H and Future Farmers of America, and subsequently, they take over the family farm. Now their inheritance and their future are gone, often resulting in resentment and the blaming of their parents for mismanagement. In a small town in North Dakota there were 14 suicides of people living on farms in 14 months, and teenage alcoholism is rising rapidly. In Nebraska one minister reported a tripling in the number of suicide calls he had received over the previous year. In Iowa, Youth and

Shelter Services reported a sharp jump in rural teenage runaways (Wall, 1985).

Another group, while small in number, appears to need additional attention: rural veterans. While most veterans gravitate toward urban areas where Veterans Administration services are more plentiful, veterans remain visible in rural areas and in great need of additional support and counseling. A study of the homeless in Vermont found "homeless veterans who seem to be making rounds from V.A. hospital to V.A. hospital around New England" (Vermont Department of Human Services, 1985).

CONCLUSION

The continuing rural economic crisis ensures that homelessness will remain a problem in rural America. For the most part, it is the working poor and farm families who are the newest rural homeless. Compared with their urban counterparts, they are younger; live in intact, two-parent, two-worker families; and have strong ties to their local community but few economic prospects. They disproportionately live in states that discriminate against intact families in their assistance programs and in communities dominated by a single industry in distress, where their only alternative is a minimum wage, service sector job.

They often face two equally unpleasant options: moving in with friends or relatives or moving in search of employment. In either case, in the long term, they are plagued by the lack of low-cost, affordable housing. Even when subsidized public housing is available, it is generally in the larger rural towns and seldom in the smaller communities that many rural homeless would prefer. Regardless of location, waiting lists for subsidized housing can stretch for years.

The health status of the rural homeless and their utilization of services do not appear to be significantly different from those for the urban homeless. Malnutrition, alcoholism and substance abuse, dental problems, stress, depression, and mental illness are pervasive. Many infants and children suffer from a failure to thrive, malnutrition, and accidents, while teenagers also face high rates of venereal disease and pregnancy, often without the benefit of prenatal care.

In times of emergency, access to physical health care appears adequate. By contrast, routine or preventive care services are seldom sought because of significant barriers to access, shame, or hostility toward the health care system.

Because of the importance of overcoming barriers to routine and preventive care, outreach efforts by community health centers would appear to be critical. As one HHS regional administrator noted, community health centers are the "backbone" of the health care delivery system in the poorest counties. Yet, the centers are being pushed in what appears to be incompatible directions. The long-term strategy of increasing their income from paying patients appears to be difficult to reconcile with the centers' original mission of meeting the needs of the poor and underserved.

The dramatic changes now taking place in farming communities, particularly within the families of financially distressed farmers, are reminiscent of the self-blame, depression, and suicidal tendencies seen in the 1930s. Farm communities seem to be splintering, providing little sympathy or support for neighbors in economic distress. These farm families then tend to turn inward, using few support services such as shelters or mental health networks. Enhanced outreach efforts such as those provided by the Agriculture Extension Service, child protection, workers, or innovative programs such as the peer counseling program cited earlier appear warranted in an effort to break this unhealthy, self-imposed isolation.

State mental health institutions in rural areas have recently begun to cooperate more extensively with community shelters that accept the chronically mentally ill. Simple efforts at coordinating discharge planning can be of great importance, as demonstrated by the Fargo, North Dakota, shelter.

In the course of site visits, a number of homeless farm families communicated their belief that income support programs—in particular, food stamps—used eligibility criteria that systematically disqualified farmers from receiving timely assistance that might have forestalled their descent into homelessness. Several social workers affirmed this claim. This suggests that there is a need for a systematic assessment of food stamp and other income support programs to determine whether better targeting of these existing programs could serve as an important preventive measure.

Finally, there is a need for additional research on the rural homeless and their health care needs. Two reports that are now under way may be helpful. The Housing Assistance Council is conducting a survey of community action agencies that have been active in working with the rural homeless. The National Coalition for the Homeless is also at work on a report on rural homelessness in the South and is conducting more extensive site visits than those used to prepare this appendix. Both studies should be available in the fall of 1988.

A more systematic assessment of the health care needs of the rural homeless in areas served by the federally funded community and migrant health centers would appear to be a logical starting point for future data collection.

REFERENCES

Brown, D. L., and K. L. Deavers. No date. The Changing of the Rural and Economic Demographic Situation in the Eighties. Washington, D.C.: U.S. Department of Agriculture Economic Research Service. (Unpublished draft.)

California Department of Economic Opportunity. 1986. The Status of Poverty in California, 1984–1985: A Report by the Advisory Commission. Sacramento: California Department of Economic Opportunity.

Congressional Research Service. 1986. Rural hospitals and Medicare's Prospective Payment System. A background paper prepared for use by the members of the Senate Committee on Finance. Washington, D.C.: Congressional Research Service.

Elison, G. No date. Frontier areas: Problem for delivery of health care services. Rural Health Care: The Newsletter of the National Rural Health Association 8(5):1.

Food Research and Action Council. 1987. Miles to Go: Barriers to Participation by the Rural Poor in the Federal Food Assistance Programs. Washington, D.C.: The Food Research and Action Council.

Frank, R., and C. L. Streeter. 1987. The bitter harvest: The question of homelessness in rural America. Pp. 36–45 in Social Work in Rural Areas: Proceedings of the Tenth National Institute on Social Work in Rural Areas, A. Summers, J. M. Schriver, P. Sundet, and R. Meinert, eds. Batesville: Arkansas College of Social Work Program.

Ghelfi, L. 1986. Poverty Among Black Families in the Nonmetro South. Rural Development Research Report no. 62. Washington, D.C.: Economic Research Service, U.S. Department of Agriculture.

Heffernen, J. B., and W. D. Heffernen. 1986. When farming families have to give up farming. Rural Development Perspectives 2(June):18.

Hoppe, R. A. 1985. Economic Structure and Change in Persistently Low-Income Nonmetro Counties. Rural Development Research Report no. 50. Washington, D.C.: Economic Research Service, U.S. Department of Agriculture.

Housing Assistance Council. 1984. Taking Stock: Rural People and Poverty from 1970 to 1983. Washington, D.C.: Housing Assistance Council.

Kindig, D., and H. Movassaghi. 1987. Physician supply: Small rural areas falling behind. Rural Health Care: The Newsletter of the National Rural Health Association 9(5):10.

Mariani, D. 1987. First Water Campground: Demographic Analysis. Flagstaff: Northern Arizona University. (Unpublished.)

Maryland Department of Human Resources. 1986. Where Do You Go from Nowhere: Homelessness in Maryland. Annapolis: Maryland Department of Human Resources.

McCormick, B. 1987. Economics, lack of services, thwart rural psychiatric care delivery. AMA News, May 4: 6.

National Association of Community Health Centers. 1987. Rural Health Policy Statement. Washington, D.C.: National Association of Community Mental Health Centers.

Ohio Department of Mental Health. 1985. Homelessness in Ohio: A Study of People in Need. Columbus: Ohio Department of Mental Health.

Ranney, R. J. 1986. Rural health crisis: The effects of the rural economy on primary health care. Pp. 53–64 in Children and Families in the Midwest: Employment, Family Services and the Rural Economy. Select Committee on Children, Youth and Families, U.S. Congress, House of Representatives. Washington, D.C.: U.S. Government Printing Office.

Redburn, F. S., and T. F. Buss. 1987. Responding to America's Homeless: Public Policy Alternatives. New York: Praeger.

Sinclair, W. 1987. Grief is growing on farm land. The Washington Post, May 24: A3.

Southern Minnesota Family Farm Fund. 1986. Questionnaire. Albert Lea, Minnesota: Southern Minnesota Family Farm Fund.

U.S. Congress, Senate, Committee on Finance. 1986. P. 77 in Hearing of the U.S. Senate Committee on Finance: Examination of Rural Hospitals Under the Medicare Program. Washington, D.C.: U.S. Government Printing Office.

U.S. Congress, Senate, Committee on Governmental Affairs. 1986. P. 1 in Governing the Heartland: Can Rural Communities Survive the Farm Crisis? Washington, D.C.: U.S. Government Printing Office.

Vermont Department of Human Services. 1985. Homelessness in Vermont. Montpelier: Vermont Department of Human Services.

Wall, W. 1985. Growing up afraid: Farm crisis is taking subtle toll on children. The Wall Street Journal, November 7: 1.

Wilson, H. 1983. Housing Assistance Council Testimony: The Rural Homeless. Washington, D.C.: Housing Assistance Council.

D

Site Visits and Meetings with Local Providers of Services to the Homeless

As part of the research plan for this study, members of the committee and members of the study staff conducted site visits to various programs serving the homeless in 11 cities: Boston; Chicago; Kansas City; Lexington; Los Angeles; Milwaukee; Nashville; San Diego; San Francisco; St. Louis; and Washington, D.C. In addition, site visits to observe the problems of homeless people in rural areas were conducted under special funding from the U.S. Department of Health and Human Services in Alabama, Minnesota, Mississippi, and North Dakota. In those cities that received grants from the Health Care for the Homeless program jointly funded by the Robert Wood Johnson Foundation and the Pew Memorial Trust (Johnson-Pew HCH), the sites visited were primarily those connected with this program.

The following sites were visited:

The Cardinal Medeiros Day Center of the Kit Clarke Senior House (Boston): A day program for the elderly homeless that operates an outreach van throughout Boston; in addition to serving food to the elderly homeless, the van is staffed by a nurse who visually observes the homeless people for signs of illness or medical problems.

Christ Church (St. Louis): A shelter for homeless adults and homeless families located in a church-owned building; the shelter provides health evaluation and education through the services of a public health nurse.

Christ House (Washington, D.C.): A 34-bed convalescent center for homeless people with medical problems; located in a restored apartment building, this facility includes a full medical and nursing clinic and on-site living quarters for the medical staff.

City Union Mission (Kansas City): A shelter, a transitional living program, and

218

an alcohol detoxification program for homeless men; the facility has an on-site nursing clinic.

Cook County Jail (Chicago): A prison with a highly regarded medical program; since some homeless people receive medical care only if they are incarcerated, this facility was toured to observe the quality of such care.

Cooper's Place (Chicago): A drop-in center for homeless men; health screening services are provided by the Chicago Johnson-Pew Health Care for the Homeless project.

Downtown Clinic (Nashville): A central clinic operated under the Nashville Johnson-Pew HCH project; this is the first HCH project to be incorporated into an existing governmental structure and is now operating as a public clinic of the city and county health department.

Emergency Lodge (Kansas City): A shelter operated by the Salvation Army that serves both individual adults and homeless families; this program also has a transitional living apartment project for homeless families.

Emergency Lodge (Milwaukee): Also operated by the Salvation Army; this program for individual adults and families receives health screening services from the Milwaukee Johnson-Pew HCH project and health care services from a nearby community health center.

Emergency Lodge (St. Louis): Operated by the Salvation Army, this shelter serves homeless families; its program includes a day care center for children so that their parents can search for employment or vocational training during the day.

Family Crisis Center (Milwaukee): A shelter for single-parent families that provides a broad spectrum of social service programs; it receives health care services from the Milwaukee Johnson-Pew HCH project.

Firehouse Annex (Chicago): A day center and transitional living program for homeless women; it receives health screening services from the Chicago Johnson-Pew HCH project.

Folsom Street Hotel (San Francisco): The site of a supportive living program for homeless people with acquired immune deficiency syndrome (AIDS) administered by Catholic Charities.

Guest House (Milwaukee): A shelter for individual adults with a high prevalence of mental illness among its client population; it receives health care services from the Milwaukee Johnson-Pew HCH project and mental health assessments from the county hospital.

Harbor House (St. Louis): A three-stage (detoxification, maintenance of sobriety, and reintegration into the community) alcohol rehabilitation program for homeless men; along with Harbor Light, a shelter for homeless men located adjacent to it, this program is operated by the Salvation Army.

Horizon Center for the Homeless (Lexington): A day center for homeless adults with a nursing clinic operated in conjunction with the College of Nursing of the University of Kentucky.

Hospitality House (St. Louis): A shelter for homeless adults, primarily women; it receives health care services from a public health nurse and a nearby health clinic.

House of Ruth (Washington, D.C.): A multisite program for homeless women, including shelters for battered women and homeless women who are pregnant; it receives health care services from the Washington Johnson-Pew HCH project.

Larkin Street Youth Center (San Francisco): A day center for homeless runaway and throwaway youths; the center has a health clinic, a group counseling program, and an aggressive AIDS prevention education program.

Lemuel Shattuck Hospital (Jamaica Plains, Mass.): The site of a 20-bed convalescent program located within a municipal shelter that is part of a state health care facility, but funded by the Boston Johnson-Pew HCH project.

Life Ministries (San Diego): A mission shelter for homeless men that operates an on-site all-volunteer medical and nursing clinic in the evenings.

Long Island Shelter (Boston): A municipal shelter for the homeless with an on-site nursing clinic.

Meharry Community Mental Health Center (Nashville): A community mental health center that provides mental health workers to the Nashville Johnson-Pew HCH project to conduct street outreach to the homeless mentally ill.

Near North Health Center Outpost Clinic (Chicago): A community health center that serves as one of the sites for the Chicago Johnson-Pew HCH project's mobile team.

Oakland Independence Support Center (Oakland, Calif.): A self-help day program operated by and for people with histories of psychiatric hospitalization; the center provides assistance in locating affordable housing for members who are or may become homeless.

Pilgrim House (Kansas City): A shelter for homeless families operated as part of the City Union Mission; Pilgrim House receives health and social services from the Kansas City project for health care for homeless people, which was developed as a result of public and private effort when Kansas City did not receive one of the Johnson-Pew HCH project grants.

Pine Street Inn (Boston): One of the oldest shelters for homeless men in the United States; the Inn has its own medical and nursing clinic, as well as a separate clinic operated by the Boston Johnson-Pew HCH project.

Project Hope (Boston): A shelter for homeless families that receives health services from the Boston Johnson-Pew HCH project's family health team.

Restart, Inc. (Kansas City): An interfaith transitional living program (which also provides emergency shelter during periods of weather extremes); this program places a heavy emphasis on vocational and social services, including a revolving fund to provide financial assistance to homeless people starting their own businesses.

So Others Might Eat (SOME) (Washington, D.C.): A soup kitchen that also provides an array of medical, dental, and support services to homeless people.

Shamrock Club (St. Louis): A membership day center for mentally ill homeless adults; receives health care services from a nearby health clinic.

St. Anthony's Clinic (San Francisco): One of the oldest health care programs serving homeless people in the United States; the clinic is divided into two halves, one serving individual adults and the other serving families.

St. Benedict's Meal Site (Milwaukee): An evening meal program that serves between 500 and 700 meals per night; an on-site clinic is operated by the Milwaukee Johnson-Pew HCH project 2 nights per week.

St. Francis House (Boston): A multiservice center for homeless adult men and women; it has a health clinic (partly funded by the Boston Johnson-Pew HCH project) and mental health and vocational training programs.

Union Rescue Mission (Los Angeles): A shelter for homeless men located in the skid row section of Los Angeles; it is the site for a nursing clinic funded by the Los Angeles Johnson-Pew HCH project.

Union Rescue Mission (Nashville): A large shelter for homeless men with its own medical and dental clinics primarily staffed by volunteer doctors and dentists and students from Meharry Medical School and Meharry College of Dentistry.

Valley Shelter, Inc. (Los Angeles): A shelter for homeless adults and families located in a former motel in the San Fernando Valley section of Los Angeles County; it receives health, mental health, and social services from the Los Angeles Johnson-Pew HCH project.

Venice Family Clinic (Los Angeles): A free clinic founded in the 1960s; it receives funding from the Los Angeles Johnson-Pew HCH project to provide health care to homeless families in the Venice Beach/Santa Monica area.

Veterans Administration Community Residence Program (Lexington): One of many such programs operated by the U.S. Veterans Administration, this program places physically and/or mentally disabled veterans into residential programs at the time of their discharge from a VA medical center as a means of preventing them from becoming homeless.

Veterans Administration Outreach Program (St. Louis): One of several programs initiated as a result of legislative action in the winter of 1986–1987; this program sends outreach workers onto the streets to identify homeless veterans in an attempt to bring them into the VA system for services.

YWCA (San Diego): A program to provide temporary housing to chronically ill homeless women via contract with the Division of Mental Health Services of the San Diego County Department of Health Services.

In addition to these sites that were visited, members of the committee and the study staff met with the following groups of local officials and service providers:

- Congressman Bill Boner (now mayor of Nashville, Tennessee), April 20, 1987.
- Kansas City Health Care for the Homeless People staff, April 30, 1987.
- Lexington, Kentucky, city officials and not-for-profit service providers, April 21, 1987.
- Los Angeles County Department of Health, May 6, 1987.
- Los Angeles County Department of Mental Health, May 6, 1987.
- Los Angeles Health Care for the Homeless Project Governance Committee, May 5, 1987.

- National Street Outreach Conference, Milwaukee, April 28, 1987.
- San Diego (City) director of Community Services, May 4, 1987.
- San Diego (County) Department of Health Services, May 4, 1987.
- San Diego (County) Department of Health Service, Division of Mental Health Services, Central Region, May 4, 1987.
- San Francisco AIDS Advisory Committee, May 8, 1987.
- San Francisco City/County Human Rights Commission AIDS discrimination specialist, May 8, 1987.
- San Francisco Homeless Service Providers' Coalition, May 7, 1987.
- San Francisco Joint Task Force on Homeless Veterans, May 8, 1987.
- St. Louis Health Care for the Homeless Coalition, May 1, 1987.
- St. Thomas Hospital, Nashville, Tennessee, April 20, 1987.
- Tennessee Association of Primary Care Centers, Nashville, Tennessee, April 20, 1987.

E Acknowledgments

Throughout this study, the committee and its staff have been assisted immeasurably by numerous organizations and individuals. The committee and staff wish to gratefully acknowledge their assistance. We apologize to anyone we have inadvertently omitted.

WILLIAM BONER, Mayor, Nashville, Tenn.
PHILIP BRICKNER, St. Vincent's Hospital and Medical Center, New York City
KAREN CARNEY, Health Care for the Homeless Program, Birmingham, Ala.
MARTIN COHEN, Robert Wood Johnson Foundation Program for the Chronic Mentally Ill, Boston, Mass.
MICHAEL COUSINEAU, Health Care for the Homeless Program, Los Angeles, Calif.
PAUL ERRERA, U.S. Veterans Administration, Washington, D.C.
PAMELA FISCHER, The Johns Hopkins University
DAVID FLANDERS, U.S. House of Representatives staff, Washington, D.C.
ROBERT GAINS, U.S. Veterans Administration, Washington, D.C.
HOPE GLEICHER, Health Care for the Homeless of Baltimore City, Baltimore, Md.
JANELLE GOETSCHEUS, Christ House, Washington, D.C.
HELEN HALLINAN, United Hospital Fund of New York, New York City
THOMAS HICKEY, Health Care for the Homeless Program, Milwaukee, Wis.

ROBERT KRAUSE, U.S. Veterans Administration, Lexington, Ky.

IRENE SHIFREN LEVINE, National Institute of Mental Health, Rockville, Md.

ADA LINDSAY, University of California at Los Angeles

JOHN LOZIER, Health Care for the Homeless Program, Nashville, Tenn.

BARBARA LUBRAN, National Institute of Alcoholism and Alcohol Abuse, Rockville, Md.

MAX MICHAEL, Health Care for the Homeless Program, Birmingham, Ala.

SUSAN NEIBACHER, United Hospital Fund, New York City

ANN PARKER, Horizon Center, Lexington, Ky.

ROBERT PRENTICE, Health Care for the Homeless Program, San Francisco, Calif.

THOMAS PRZYBECK, Washington University

KEITH RADCLIFFE, Health Care for the Homeless Program, Boston, Mass.

LEE ROBINS, Washington University

JEAN SUMMERFIELD, Health Care for the Homeless Program, Chicago, Ill.

HAROLD TATTEN, University of California at Los Angeles

CLEONICE TAVANI, U.S. Department of Health and Human Services, Rockville, Md.

ROBERT WALKINGTON, U.S. Department of Health and Human Services, Rockville, Md.

JUDY WEILEPP, Health Care for the Homeless Coalition, St. Louis, Mo.

MARILYN WILLIAMS, Truman Medical Center, Kansas City, Mo.

STEVEN WOBIDO, Robert Wood Johnson Foundation-Pew Memorial Trust Health Care for the Homeless Program, New York City

JAMES D. WRIGHT, Social and Demographic Research Institute, Amherst, Mass.

F Biographical Notes on Committee Members

DREW ALTMAN, Ph.D., is commissioner of the New Jersey Department of Human Services. He came to his post in 1986 from a position as vice president of the Robert Wood Johnson Foundation. Prior to that, Dr. Altman held an administrative position with the Health Care Financing Administration at the U.S. Department of Health and Human Services.

ELLEN L. BASSUK, M.D., is associate professor of psychiatry at Harvard Medical School. She has completed various research studies and written extensively about the origins of homelessness, the needs of homeless families, and the impact of homelessness on children. In 1988 she became president of The Better Homes Foundation in Chestnut Hill, Massachusetts, a new organization created to help homeless families.

WILLIAM R. BREAKEY, M.D., is currently the director of the Community Psychiatry Program at the Johns Hopkins School of Medicine as well as associate professor in the Department of Psychiatry and Behavioral Sciences. He has carried out research on homeless persons suffering from mental illness and alcohol problems and has provided clinical care for them.

A. ALAN FISCHER, M.D., is professor and founding chairman of the Department of Family Medicine at the Indiana University School of Medicine. A practicing family physician since 1953, Dr. Fischer is active in educating students and young physicians to meet people's primary health care needs.

225

CHARLES R. HALPERN is professor of law at the City University of New York Law School at Queens College and senior fellow at Yale Law School. He was the founding dean of the CUNY Law School and the cofounder of the Mental Health Law Project and the Center for Law and Social Policy. He has been actively involved in efforts to define and protect the legal rights of mentally impaired people.

JUDITH R. LAVE, Ph.D., has been a faculty member at Carnegie Mellon University; director of the Division of Economic and Quantitative Analysis, Office of the Deputy Assistant Secretary for Planning and Evaluation, Department of Health and Human Services; and director of the Office of Research in the Health Care Financing Administration. She is currently professor of health economics at the Graduate School of Public Health, University of Pittsburgh.

JACK A. MEYER is founder and president of New Directions for Policy, a research and policy organization that develops, analyzes, and evaluates social policies for government, business, and the foundation community. Mr. Meyer is the author of numerous books on health care policy. He is currently serving as a senior consultant to the Ford Foundation's Project on Social Welfare and the American Future.

GLORIA R. SMITH, R.N., Ph.D., is presently dean and professor of nursing at Wayne State University College of Nursing in Detroit; during her service on the study committee, she was the State Health Director for Michigan. Prior to that Dr. Smith was dean and professor at the University of Oklahoma College of Nursing (Health Sciences Center) in Oklahoma City.

LOUISA R. STARK, Ph.D., is an adjunct professor in the Department of Anthropology at Arizona State University. She was formerly professor of anthropology at the University of Wisconsin and has served as director of anthropology at the Heard Museum in Phoenix. Dr. Stark serves on the Salvation Army Social Services Advisory Board and, since 1984, has been president of the National Coalition for the Homeless.

NATHAN J. STARK, a lawyer, is senior vice chancellor emeritus for Health Sciences, University of Pittsburgh, and president emeritus of the University Health Center of Pittsburgh. He served as undersecretary of the U.S. Department of Health and Human Services in 1979–1980.

MARVIN TURCK, M.D., is professor of medicine, University of Washington School of Medicine. During his service on the study committee he also held the posts of medical director of Harborview Medical Center and associate dean of the University of Washington School of Medicine. Dr. Turck is editor of the *Journal of Infectious Diseases*.

BRUCE C. VLADECK is president of the United Hospital Fund of New York. He also serves as a member of the Prospective Payment Assessment Commission, the Board of Directors of the New York City Health and Hospitals Corporation, and the New York State Advisory Council on Graduate Medical Education. Before joining the United Hospital Fund in 1983, Dr. Vladeck held positions at the Robert Wood Johnson Foundation, the New Jersey State Department of Health, and Columbia University.

PHYLLIS B. WOLFE, M.S.W., A.C.S.W., developed a prototype mental health care program for the homeless in Washington, D.C., and was its project director from 1981 to 1985. In 1984–1985 she designed and implemented the Public–Private Partnership Health Care for the Homeless Demonstration Project in Washington, D.C., sponsored by the Robert Wood Johnson Foundation and the Pew Memorial Trust; she continues to serve the Project as its executive director.

Index